ANESTHESIOLOGY

National Medical Series for Independent Study

NMS
CLINICAL MANUALS

ANESTHESIOLOGY

Randall S. Glidden, M.D.

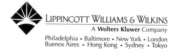

LIPPINCOTT WILLIAMS & WILKINS
A **Wolters Kluwer** Company

Philadelphia · Baltimore · New York · London
Buenos Aires · Hong Kong · Sydney · Tokyo

Editor: Neil Marquardt
Managing Editor: Beth Goldner
Marketing Manager: Scott Lavine
Production Editor: Christina Remsberg
Compositor: In House Composition
Printer: Data Reproductions

Library of Congress Cataloging-in-Publication Data

Library of Congress data has been applied for and is available.

The publishers have made every effort to trace the copyright holders for borrowed material. If they have inadvertently overlooked any, they will be pleased to make the necessary arrangements at the first opportunity.

To purchase additional copies of this book call our customer service department at **(800) 638-3030** or fax orders to **(301) 824-7390**. International customers should call **(301) 714-2324.**

Visit Lippincott Williams & Wilkins on the Internet: http://www.lww.com. Lippincott Williams & Wilkins customer service representatives are available from 8:30 am to 6:00 pm, EST.

03 04 05

1 2 3 4 5 6 7 8 9 10

CONTRIBUTORS

Sheila R. Barnett, M.D.
Assistant Professor
Department of Anesthesia and Critical Care
Harvard Medical School
Beth Israel Deaconess Medical Center
Boston, MA

Robert I. Cohen, M.D.
Instructor in Anesthesia
Anesthesiologist and Pain Physician
Department of Anesthesia and Critical Care
Harvard Medical School
Beth Israel Deaconess Medical Center
Boston, MA

Stephen A. Cohen, M.D., M.B.A.
Director, Industry Relations
Department of Anesthesia and Critical Care
Beth Israel Deaconess Medical Center
Boston, MA

Mark E. Comunale, M.D.
Associate Professor
Department of Anesthesia and Critical Care
Harvard Medical School
Beth Israel Deaconess Medical Center
Boston, MA

David C. Lai, M.D.
Coordinator of Resident Curriculum
Department of Anesthesia and Critical Care
Harvard Medical School
Beth Israel Deaconess Medical Center
Boston, MA

Lisa L. Lombard, M.D.
Instructor in Anesthesia
Department of Anesthesia and Critical Care
Harvard Medical School
Beth Israel Deaconess Medical Center
Boston, MA

Selina A. Long, M.D.
Attending Anesthesiologist
Department of Anesthesia and Critical Care
Harvard Medical School
Beth Israel Deaconess Medical Center
Boston, MA

John S. Mashikian, M.D.
Director, Division of Cardiac Anesthesia
Beth Israel Deaconess Medical Center
Boston, MA

Jyotsna Nagda, M.D.
Instructor in Anesthesia
Department of Anesthesia and Critical Care
Harvard Medical School
Beth Israel Deaconess Medical Center
Boston, MA

Samir K. Patel, M.D.
Instructor in Anesthesia
Program Director, Critical Care Fellowship
Department of Anesthesia and Critical Care
Harvard Medical School
Beth Israel Deaconess Medical Center
Boston, MA

Stephen Pratt, M.D.
Instructor in Anesthesia
Department of Anesthesia and Critical Care
Harvard Medical School
Beth Israel Deaconess Medical Center
Boston, MA

Christopher Quartararo, M.D.
Instructor in Anesthesia
Department of Anesthesia and Critical Care
Harvard Medical School
Beth Israel Deaconess Medical Center
Boston, MA

Daniel Talmor, M.D.
Instructor in Anesthesia
Department of Anesthesia and Critical Care
Harvard Medical School
Beth Israel Deaconess Medical Center
Boston, MA

Mary Ann Vann, M.D.
Instructor in Anesthesia
Department of Anesthesia and Critical Care
Harvard Medical School
Beth Israel Deaconess Medical Center
Boston, MA

DEDICATION

For Steve

CONTENTS

FOREWORD

NMS Clinical Manual of Anesthesiology is a practical tour guide through the scientific world of the anesthesiologist. Dr. Glidden and his coauthors skillfully guide students through the clinical activity and scientific reasoning behind those activities that anesthesiologists carry out every day as they care for their patients. Medical students arrive at their initial exposure to the specialty of anesthesiology after having learned chemistry, physics, organic chemistry, physiology, anatomy, and pathophysiology. Yet when they first encounter the specialty of anesthesiology, their attention is often so focused on mastering the practical skills of placing IVs or intubating the trachea that they miss how their hard-earned fund of basic science knowledge relates to this specialty. This handbook helps connect the clinical practice of the anesthesiologist to the scientific foundation behind that practice. This book, step by step, walks the student through the practice and science of this specialty.

The book starts with an historical perspective—what life was like before the discovery of anesthesia. Both the patient and physician suffered—for most of us, surgery without anesthesia is unimaginable. The trip from the time before anesthesia all the way to our current-day molecular understanding of pain pathways is difficult to capture in a brief medical school clerkship, in a chapter, or even in a book. However, this is exactly what Dr. Glidden has achieved as he takes us from the history of anesthesia to the place of anesthesia in modern medicine.

The framework of the rest of the book allows the reader to first see, in overview, the orderly steps of a "simple anesthetic." It then incorporates the basic sciences of pharmacology and physiology to put it all together so we can understand the details of a complex, although exceedingly common, "anesthesia case study." The pharmacology of anesthetic techniques is presented in four clear chapters, which cover inhaled anesthetics, intravenous anesthetics, local anesthetics, and the range of medications that are used for sedation. These pharmacologic agents are the primary tools of the anesthesiologist. The next six chapters cover the physiology and pathophysiology of the anesthetic patient. As Julie M. Fenster recounted in the book *Ether Day,* the field of anesthesiology has its roots in chemistry. To quote my daughter's chemistry teacher, Mr. McGillicuddy, "We are the chemists of the human body." The anesthesiologist must understand both the pharmacology of the agents they use and have a facile knowledge of the human body, and its physiology and pathophysiology. To put it all together requires facility with all the systems of the human body. When Harvard Medical School adopted small group tutorials as the basis of its preclinical education, faculties from all departments were recruited to lead the tutorial, generally in their own specialties. Over the years, I have participated in many of these courses, including renal, cardiovascular, and respiratory physiology as well as hematology and gastroenterology. When asked by a colleague how could I teach so many different specialties I replied that, "as an anesthesiologist I have to deal with all those systems and if I was not expert in each my patient would surely suffer." Anesthesiologists are practicing physiologists and pharmacologists; this book helps make that breadth of the field clear.

The final section of the book highlights four of the subspecialties of anesthesia, including ambulatory, cardiac, and obstetric anesthesia as well as pain management. These chapters provide an often unseen view of the depth of understanding that comes with a more narrow focus on one subspecialty. From understanding the vascular reactivity of the placental vessels (critical for safely practicing obstetric anesthesia) to developing the skill to perform and interpret transesophageal echocardiography (a critical new development that helps the cardiac anesthesiologist evaluate both right and left ventricular function in their patients under anesthesia), the range of subspecialty anesthesia is well represented. The four subspecialties in this book give the student a perspective from which to imagine what the other subspecialties might be like, such as anesthesia for pediatrics patients, anesthesia for neurosurgery, or the fascinating issues of anesthesia for the patient undergoing magnetic resonance imaging (just how do you take that big metal anesthesia machine into a room with a magnet that size?). As medical science grows, so too do the tools and challenges for the anesthesiologist.

This book presents the practice of anesthesia so that the student can look past the challenge of the dexterity needed to perform invasive procedures to the deeply intellectual challenge of learning how to control human physiology during the trauma of surgery and severe pain. It is an important companion to any introductory anesthesia experience, and will ensure that even the medical student who does not plan to become an anesthesiologist will understand more about the field than just its procedures.

The human body has evolved over millions of years and has developed exquisitely sensitive reflexes to help it survive injury, whether from a saber tooth tiger or a surgeon's knife. The job of the anesthesiologist is to understand and control these powerful reflexes and with vigilant attention to detail and a broad base of knowledge, safely and with as little pain as possible carry the patient through the trauma of surgery, maintain homeostasis, and then bring the patient back to normal preoperative functioning. This book gives students insight into the art and the science of anesthesia.

Nancy E. Oriol, M.D.
Associate Dean of Student Affairs
Harvard Medical School

PREFACE

A medical student beginning the usual 1–2 week anesthesiology clerkship faces a daunting task: how does one tackle the vast knowledge base of a medical specialty whose major textbook (Miller's *Anesthesia*) is 500 pages longer than the venerable *Cecil Textbook of Medicine?** Such a brief clinical exposure demands a textbook that provides the student with the basics of the practice, covers the key concepts of this specialty that every student should know prior to graduation from medical school, and is written in a format and length that the student can read and digest in a short time period. We wrote this handbook with these requirements clearly in mind.

Part I, Perioperative Anesthesia Care, comprises the largest portion of the book and covers topics such as pharmacology of anesthetic drugs, airway management, preoperative evaluation, and other key chapters that focus on the anesthetic care of the surgical patient. Case studies at the beginning and end of Part I help solidify the concepts presented in these chapters.

In Part II, Anesthesiology Specialty Areas, chapters on ambulatory, obstetric, and cardiac anesthesia, and acute and chronic pain management cover some of the most important subspecialty areas of anesthesiology. These chapters give the student a notion of the depth and breadth of 21st century anesthesiology and should provide further reinforcement of many of the anesthesia concepts discussed in Part I.

Throughout this handbook we have tried to write the chapters clearly, concisely, and with enough detail to adequately cover the topics without burdening the reader with excessive minutia. Suggested readings at the end of each chapter allow the student with more time or interest to "dig deeper" if desired. All of the authors are experienced anesthesiologists who share a commitment to medical student education as well as to safe and competent patient care. We have written this handbook for all students of anesthesiology. We hope that you will find it a useful companion to your anesthesiology clinical activities and that it will find its way into the back pocket of many a scrub suit.

Randall S. Glidden, M.D.

Cecil Textbook of Medicine, 21st edition, 2000, 2308 pages; Miller *Anesthesia,* 5th edition, 2000, 2877 pages.

ACKNOWLEDGMENTS

I am grateful to Holly P. Glidden for her moral support and editing skills, and to both Elizabeth Nieginski and Beth Goldner at Lippincott Williams & Wilkins for their professional assistance during the planning and editing phases of this book. I also thank our Chairman, Dr. Carol Warfield, who gave her advice and encouragement, the contributing authors who made this book possible, and the students who inspired its writing.

CHAPTER 1

Introduction:
Anesthesiology Past and Present

Randall S. Glidden, MD

A HISTORIC SKETCH

Imagine how Gilbert Abbott, a 21-year-old painter from Boston, felt about the prospects of having surgery on the morning of October 16, 1846. Despite the fact that the operation would be performed at the famous Massachusetts General Hospital by the equally famous Harvard Professor and Chief of Surgery, John Collins Warren, Mr. Abbott must have felt rather unsettled about having the large vascular tumor removed from the left side of his neck. He was no doubt aware that the operation would require the services of several burley orderlies whose responsibility it would be to restrain him while Dr. Warren excised the neck mass as quickly as possible without the benefit of anything to relieve the incredible pain that such a procedure was sure to produce. With luck, he might have thought, the pain would be severe enough to induce a faint that would temporarily render him unaware of the excruciating trauma he was experiencing. Surgery in the mid-19th century was without doubt a nightmare for the patients as well as the surgeons.

Probably unbeknownst to Gilbert Abbott, a Boston dentist by the name of William T.G. Morton had a few days earlier announced to Dr. Warren that he had "invented" a preparation that he felt could be used to render a person insensible to the painful effects of surgery. Dr. Morton had, in fact, used a handkerchief soaked with diethyl ether to extract the tooth of one Eben Frost just two weeks before Abbott's surgery. Dr. Warren, then 68 years old and close to retirement, decided to take Morton up on his offer, inviting him "to administer to a patient who is then operated upon, the preparation which [he had] invented to diminish the sensibility of pain."

We should assume that Warren was probably a bit skeptical of Morton's "invention," since another dentist, Horace Wells, had some months earlier claimed that he could painlessly pull teeth while patients were under the influence of inhaled nitrous oxide. His attempted public demonstration of this—before Dr. Warren and a large and presumably rowdy audience of Harvard medical students—had resulted in the patient crying out in pain and Dr. Wells's nitrous oxide being declared a "humbug."

Whether skeptical or not, Dr. Warren did indeed invite Dr. Morton to use his invention on Gilbert Abbott a mere 48 hours before the scheduled surgery. Morton—who certainly must have thought a handkerchief an inappropriate delivery device for his great discovery—frantically sought the aid of Dr. Augustus Gould to design, and the instrument maker N.B. Chamberlain to craft, an apparatus suitable for ether inhalation. The now famous ether inhaler, a small glass globe fitted with valves, was constructed in the wee hours of October 16, and completed at 10 AM, which was, incidentally, the time of Mr. Abbott's surgery.

Dr. Morton arrived at the great surgical amphitheater of the Massachusetts General a full 15 minutes late, at which time the then impatient Dr. Warren reportedly remarked, "Well, Sir, your patient is ready." Morton offered some soothing words to the presumably nervous Mr. Abbott and asked that he breathe deeply from the ether apparatus. As Abbott sank into unconsciousness, Morton fired back to Warren, "Sir, *your* patient is ready!" The surgical incision and operation that followed produced little, if any, noticeably painful effects on Mr. Abbott, who said after awakening that he had only felt a scratching sensation in his neck. Dr. Warren turned to the assembled audience of hospital staff and students and said, "Gentlemen, this is no humbug."

Dr. Morton's somewhat theatrical performance was, thus, the first *public* demonstration of ether anesthesia and is commemorated every year on October 16 ("ether day") at the Massachusetts General Hospital.

But he wasn't the first. For some time before Dr. Morton's 1846 demonstration, a young physician and surgeon from Jefferson, Georgia, named Crawford Long had been quite fond of inhaling ether for its "exhilarating effects." In fact Dr. Long and many of his friends had observed that after having been under the influence of inhaled ether they would often notice the presence of "bruises and painful spots," presumably the result of some trauma received during their ether frolics. Dr. Long correctly concluded that ether had ablated the sensation of painful stimuli inflicted during its administration.

James Venable, longtime friend of Dr. Long and a frequent fellow ether inhaler, had been considering the removal of several small tumors on the back of his neck. However, as with Gilbert Abbott, the thought of that painful process gave Venable pause. Dr. Long suggested the possibility that inhalation of ether might prevent Venable's suffering during the procedure. So, on March 30, 1842, James Venable inhaled ether from a towel while Dr. Crawford Long removed one of the tumors from his neck. According to Dr. Long, after being informed that the operation was over, Venable "seemed incredulous until the tumor was shown him. He gave no evidence of suffering during the operation, and assured [Dr. Long] that he did not experience the slightest degree of pain from its performance."

Clearly Long's use of ether for surgical anesthesia predated Dr. Morton's famous anesthetic by more than 4 years. Unfortunately Dr. Long kept his discovery to himself, and only after hearing of Morton's fame in Boston did he publish his own account of ether anesthesia in December of 1849. To this day both Morton and Long are considered by most to be responsible for the introduction of ether anesthesia to the world, with preference somewhat split north and south of the Mason-Dixon line.

By the end of the nineteenth century surgical anesthesia had been universally embraced, and in 1905 a sufficiently large number of anesthesia practitioners warranted the founding of the Long Island Society of Anesthetists, which became the American Society of Anesthesiologists in 1945. Although a detailed account of the advances in anesthesiology over the ensuing century and a half is beyond the scope of this chapter, Table 1-1 summarizes some of these major events.

ANESTHESIOLOGY TODAY

Patients and surgeons alike assume that the anesthesiologist will prevent pain or suffering during surgery. The scope of the practice, of course, goes far beyond simply producing insensitivity to pain. According to the American Society of Anesthesiologists' Internet Web site (www.asahq.org/what_is_anesth.html, February 20, 2001), "anesthesiology is the practice of medicine dedicated to the relief of pain and total care of the surgical patient before, during, and after surgery." And because anesthesiologists are

Table 1-1. Some Anesthesia Milestones

Year	Event
1842	Crawford Long anesthetizes James Venable and performs first operation under ether anesthesia (not reported until 1849).
1845	Dentist Horace Wells successfully uses nitrous oxide for dental extractions; however, public demonstration fails.
1846	First public demonstration of ether anesthesia, by William T.G. Morton, in the "Ether Dome" of Massachusetts General Hospital, Boston.
1846	Oliver Wendell Holmes suggests the term "anaesthesia" to describe ether-induced state.
1847	John Snow of Great Britain publishes *On the Inhalation of the Vapour of Ether,* first anesthesia textbook.
1898	German surgeon August Bier invents spinal anesthesia using cocaine. (Administered to himself by an assistant!)
1905	Long Island Society of Anesthetists founded.
1934	Sodium thiopental introduced by Waters and Lundy.
1942	Griffith and Johnson induce surgical paralysis with curare during general anesthesia.
1950s	Halogenated inhalation anesthetics gradually replace ether.
1960s	Synthetic opioid fentanyl introduced; DeCastro and Lowenstein describe high-dose opioid anesthesia using fentanyl and morphine, respectively.
1970s	Continuous electrocardiographic monitoring becomes standard practice; invention of pulse oximeter revolutionizes patient safety; short-acting hypnotic drug propofol introduced.
1980s	Carbon dioxide and inhaled anesthetic gas monitors are routinely incorporated into anesthesia machines.
1990–2000	Anesthetic death rate falls from 1 in 10,000 to 1 in 250,000.

responsible for the nonsurgical care of the patient during the perioperative period, the term "perioperative physician" is often used to further describe the specialty.

On any given day, any patient with any disease may require any kind of operation — the anesthesiologist, therefore, must be prepared to anesthetize any such patient using not only a thorough understanding of anesthetic principles but also a broad knowledge of general medicine and the ways in which anesthetic and surgical techniques may affect the patient and his or her current medical condition during the planned surgery. The anesthesiologist must devise a perioperative plan that will take into account the patient's medical status, the planned operation, and an appropriate anesthetic, and then carry out that plan in such a way as to assure the overall safety and well-being of the patient. This is a challenging task given the current complexity of both patients and modern surgical procedures, and it requires training, skill, and diligence of practice.

Outside the operating room anesthesiologists care for patients in postanesthesia care units (PACU) and, frequently, surgical intensive care units. In addition to treating such frequent postoperative problems as pain, nausea, and hemodynamic and respiratory instability, the anesthesiologist helps assist the patient in the transition to either the surgical floor or, as is the case with the ambulatory surgery patient, the home environment.

Besides perioperative management the anesthesiologist's practice is broad: During cardiac arrests or in critically ill trauma patients, anesthesiologists often provide airway management and perform endotracheal intubation when necessary. Patients undergoing painful procedures such as cardiac catheterizations, gastrointestinal endoscopic evaluations, and electroshock therapy may have their suffering eased by sedation or anesthesia provided by anesthesiologists. Maternity patients often depend on epidural or spinal blocks administered by anesthesiologists to reduce or eliminate pain during labor. Pain centers offer a multidisciplinary approach to the management of the patient with chronic pain using the services of anesthesiologists, neurologists, psychiatrists, nurses, and physical therapists. Clearly, anesthesiologists can and do care for patients in any setting where their knowledge and expertise can be used to eliminate anxiety, discomfort, or pain.

Finally, anesthesiologists have been responsible for many advances in both clinical and basic science research. Academic anesthesiologists conduct research in nearly every medical discipline and provide for the education and training of medical students, anesthesiology residents, and nurse anesthetists.

SUMMARY

From roots dating back to the efforts by a few recreational ether users to prevent surgical suffering, anesthesiology has evolved into a challenging and indispensable medical specialty. Anesthesiologists in this country are responsible for the administration of nearly 40 million anesthetics each year, provide care to patients in the perioperative period, and participate in the treatment of many more patients outside the operating room. In addition to their clinical roles, anesthesiologists actively pursuing careers in research and education have made major contributions to their specialty and to the field of medicine in the twenty-first century. Although not every medical student will become an anesthesiologist, every medical student should be familiar with the principles of anesthesia, perioperative medicine, and safe patient care practiced by anesthesiologists.

SUGGESTED READINGS

Nuland S. The Origins of Anesthesia. The Classics of Medicine Library. Birmingham, Ala.: Gryphon Editions, 1983.

Long CW. An account of the first use of sulphuric ether by inhalation as an anaesthetic in surgical operations. South Med Surg. J 1849;5:705–713.

PART I

Perioperative Anesthetic Management

CHAPTER 2

Overview: A Simple General Anesthetic

Randall S. Glidden, MD

Of all the clinical procedures performed in modern medicine, a general anesthetic is one of the most complicated and dramatic. Anesthesiologists must use their knowledge of pharmacology and facility with anesthetic techniques to render the patient insensate to surgical pain while maintaining physiologic stability. A medical student witnessing his or her first general anesthetic can easily be overwhelmed by the anesthesiologist's actions as he skillfully takes the patient through the stages of general anesthesia. For example:

The medical student watches as the anesthesiologist, Dr. Long, wheels the patient, Mr. Morton, into the operating room and has him move onto the operating table. After attaching the appropriate monitors, Dr. Long applies an anesthesia mask to Mr. Morton's face and injects a rapid succession of drugs into the intravenous line. Within seconds Mr. Morton loses consciousness, and Dr. Long begins to ventilate his lungs by squeezing a bag attached to plastic tubing. Dr. Long turns various dials on the complicated-looking anesthesia machine. He inserts a laryngoscope into Mr. Morton's mouth and intubates his trachea. More drugs are given, more dials are turned. The surgeon places the drapes and finally starts the operation. At the end of the procedure Mr. Morton awakens from his drug-induced coma, and within minutes he is able to respond to his name by opening his eyes and then moving from the operating table back to the stretcher. Dr. Long takes him to the postanesthesia care unit (PACU), and after 2 hours Mr. Morton walks out of the hospital with his wife, apparently restored to his preanesthetized state.

Many questions run through the student's mind: What kind of anesthesia does the patient need? What drugs should be used? In what order do you give them? How do you manage the airway? How does the anesthesia machine work? How is the anesthesia maintained during the surgery? What sort of problems can arise and how do you handle them? How do you waken the patient smoothly and safely? To answer these questions the student first must understand the basic structure of a general anesthetic. This chapter will discuss the usual steps taken by anesthesiologists as they perform general anesthesia (Table 2-1). Once the medical student understands these basic steps, he or she can turn to further chapters of the book that examine general anesthesia in more detail.

Table 2-1. Steps in a Typical General Anesthetic

Step	Highlights	Average Time Required
1. Preoperative evaluation	Assessment of medical database Discussion of anesthetic choices Informed consent obtained	15–30 minutes
2. Patient preparation I (preoperative holding area)	Initial vital signs measured and "NPO" status determined Anesthetic plans confirmed Intravenous access obtained Sedation usually given	15–30 minutes
3. Patient preparation II (operating room)	Monitors attached IV patency confirmed	5–10 minutes
4. Induction of anesthesia I	Preoxygenation Intravenous induction	3–5 minutes
5. Airway management	Open airway established after loss of consciousness Insertion of LMA or ETT (if used)	2–5 minutes
6. Induction of anesthesia II	Inhalation anesthesia begun; achieve depth needed for surgery	3–10 minutes
7. Maintenance of anesthesia	Continued delivery of anesthetic agents at depth needed for surgery Indicated parameters monitored; intervention if necessary	Minutes to hours; varies with length of surgery
8. Emergence from anesthesia	Reversal of neuromuscular blockade Discontinuation of inhaled anesthetics Return of consciousness Extubation (usually)	5–15 minutes
9. Recovery from anesthesia	Vital signs and oxygenation monitored Pain management Postoperative complications treated Patient returns to preanesthetized state	1–3 hours

We will begin by taking our example patient, Mr. Morton, through his anesthetic from start to finish:

Mr. Morton is a 45-year-old man in good health who damaged the anterior cruciate ligament (ACL) of his right knee in a skiing accident. He has seen an orthopedic surgeon who has scheduled him to have an arthroscopic ACL reconstruction.

STEP 1: PREOPERATIVE EVALUATION

An anesthesiologist must evaluate every patient who is planning to have surgery requiring an anesthesiologist's care. This evaluation is often done in a preoperative clinic several days before surgery, but it can be completed on the day of surgery if the patient is healthy. During this evaluation the anesthesiologist should do the following:

1. Summarize the patient's general health, including preexisting medical conditions, allergies, and current medications.
2. Perform a brief physical examination, with focus on assessment of the airway, lungs, and cardiovascular system.
3. Discuss with the patient the anesthetic options and relative risks and benefits of each.
4. Obtain the patient's informed consent for anesthesia.
5. Provide preoperative instructions as to medications to take or avoid on the day of surgery, and when to discontinue eating and drinking (i.e., be placed "NPO," nil per os).
6. Formulate an anesthetic plan that takes into consideration the proposed surgery, the patient's medical condition, and the wishes of the patient and the surgeon.

Mr. Morton has no active medical problems, his physical examination is unremarkable, and he wishes to be "knocked out" for his surgery (rather than having regional anesthesia). He gives his informed consent for the anesthesia, and he is told not to eat or drink anything after midnight the evening before surgery.

STEP 2: PATIENT PREPARATION I (PREOPERATIVE HOLDING AREA)

Initial preoperative preparation begins with the measurement of vital signs and confirmation of NPO status. The patient then exchanges street clothes for a hospital gown. The anesthesiologist will review the anesthetic plans previously discussed in the preoperative visit to be sure the patient is in agreement. The anesthesiologist will then start an intravenous line and, if needed, any invasive monitors (e.g., arterial catheter).

Before being moved to the operating room, most patients are given an intravenous sedative, usually a short-acting benzodiazepine such as midazolam. Not only does sedation relieve some of the patient's anxiety, it often helps make the induction of anesthesia occur more smoothly.

Mr. Morton's vital signs are all normal, he has been NPO since 11:00 PM, and he still wants general anesthesia for his surgery. Dr. Long inserts a 20-gauge intravenous catheter into a vein in his left hand and gives him 2 mg of midazolam intravenously before wheeling him into the operating room.

STEP 3: PATIENT PREPARATION II (OPERATING ROOM)

After transfer into the operating room and before inducing anesthesia, the anesthesiologist will do the following:

1. Attach appropriate monitors. At a *minimum* this includes a three-lead electrocardiogram (ECG), a noninvasive blood pressure cuff, and a pulse oximeter. If invasive monitors comprise part of the anesthetic plan, they would be attached at this time as well.
2. Confirm that the intravenous line is patent and running well.

After he arrives in the operating room, Mr. Morton slides over to the operating table. Dr. Long applies the ECG leads, places a blood pressure cuff on his right arm, and attaches a pulse oximeter probe to his left index finger. He also places the leads for a neuroblockade monitor on Mr. Morton's left wrist. The intravenous line is running well.

STEP 4: INDUCTION OF ANESTHESIA I

Before the surgeon can make an incision, the patient must enter an anesthetic state in which he or she has no awareness, feeling, or response to surgical stimuli. Most anesthesiologists think of this state as a triad consisting of hypnosis (unconsciousness), amnesia, and analgesia that are provided by the anesthetic drugs. Induction usually begins with an intravenous anesthetic and then continues with an inhaled agent. The first phase of induction usually consists of the following:

1. Preoxygenation. The patient is told to breathe 100% oxygen through an anesthesia mask attached to tubing called a breathing circuit. This replaces most of the nitrogen contained in the patient's lungs with pure oxygen and lessens the chance of hypoxemia during induction.
2. Intravenous induction. Short-acting drugs such as thiopental and propofol are usually used to produce a rapid loss of consciousness.

Mr. Morton breathes deeply from the mask placed over his nose and mouth. After several deep breaths of pure oxygen, Dr. Long injects 200 mg of propofol into the intravenous port. After a few seconds, Mr. Morton no longer blinks after his eyelashes are stroked—he is unconscious.

STEP 5: AIRWAY MANAGEMENT

After the patient loses consciousness the anesthesiologist must turn his or her attention to airway management. The anesthesiologist will open the airway by lifting the chin and will then ventilate the patient's lungs by applying positive pressure by squeezing a bag attached to the breathing circuit. Once the airway is open, the induction can continue using inhaled anesthetics delivered by one of several methods:

1. Mask airway. The patient receives the inhaled anesthetic through the anesthesia mask. He will either breathe spontaneously or the anesthesiologist will assist his ventilation by applying positive pressure to the anesthesia bag.

2. Laryngeal mask airway (LMA). The LMA is a relatively new device consisting of a tube attached to an inflatable cuff. Once properly placed in the patient's posterior oropharynx, the cuff surrounds the glottic structures and provides a patent airway for ventilation. As with the mask airway, the patient can either breathe spontaneously or positive pressure can be applied.

3. Endotracheal intubation. The endotracheal tube (ETT) is usually inserted after the patient is paralyzed with a neuromuscular blocking drug. Because the cuff on the ETT seals the trachea, the ETT provides a more secure airway than the mask or the LMA. It is therefore the airway of choice if the patient is at risk for aspiration of stomach contents. The patient can breathe spontaneously, but usually a mechanical ventilator is used.

Because the operation is scheduled to take approximately 3 hours, Dr. Long believes that an ETT would be a safer choice than the mask or LMA. After Mr. Morton is unconscious Dr. Long opens his airway by lifting his chin, places the mask firmly over his nose and mouth, and applies positive pressure by squeezing the anesthesia bag. He determines that he can easily ventilate Mr. Morton's lungs, so he then injects 8 mg of vecuronium (an intermediate-acting neuromuscular blocking drug) into the intravenous catheter. After 5 minutes Dr. Long intubates Mr. Morton's trachea with ease.

STEP 6: INDUCTION OF ANESTHESIA II

Once the anesthesiologist has established an airway, an inhaled anesthetic will maintain the unconsciousness begun by the intravenous induction agent. Inhaled anesthetics offer the advantage of being safe, effective, economical, and slow to build up in the patient's body. Unlike hypnotic drugs such as propofol, inhaled anesthetics provide hypnosis, amnesia, and analgesia—all the components of the anesthetic triad in one agent. The anesthesia machine is used to mix these agents with oxygen and then deliver them safely and accurately to the breathing circuit. Inhaled agents fall into two categories:

1. Volatile anesthetics. (Examples: isoflurane, desflurane, sevoflurane.) Because they are liquids at room temperature a vaporizer is used to convert the liquids to gases and then precisely deliver them to the anesthesia breathing circuit. Volatile anesthetics can either be given alone or, more commonly, combined with nitrous oxide.

2. Nitrous oxide. This is a gas of rather low anesthetic potency and low cost that is rarely given without a volatile anesthetic. Adding nitrous oxide reduces the amount of volatile anesthetic required.

After intubation Dr. Long adjusts the dials on the anesthesia machine flowmeters to deliver 2 L of nitrous oxide and 1 L of oxygen per minute. Next he turns on the desflurane vaporizer and sets the dial to deliver a 5% concentration of desflurane vapor to the inhaled gases. He turns on the ventilator on the anesthesia machine.

STEP 7: MAINTENANCE OF ANESTHESIA

After several minutes the inhaled anesthetics the patient has been breathing will reach an equilibrium concentration in the brain that will produce a sufficient depth of anesthesia for the surgery. Once this level has been achieved the anesthetic maintenance phase has begun. This is the longest portion of an anesthetic, and the anesthesiologist usually performs the following actions:

1. Deliver inhaled anesthetic gases at levels that provide adequate depth of anesthesia for the surgical stimuli.
2. Add narcotic drugs, as needed, both to lessen the requirement for inhaled anesthetic agents and to provide analgesia during the emergence and recovery phases of anesthesia.
3. Give neuromuscular blocking drugs to maintain muscle paralysis if required.
4. Give other adjunctive drugs if indicated (e.g., antiemetic agents).
5. Follow all monitored parameters and intervene when necessary.

Mr. Morton's knee has been prepped and draped by the surgical team. Dr. Long sees that the anesthetic agent analyzer indicates that the gas concentrations of desflurane and nitrous oxide have reached levels appropriate for the surgery. All of Mr. Morton's vital signs are within his usual normal limits, and they stay in that range for the rest of the procedure. One hour before the end of the surgery, Dr. Long gives more fentanyl in anticipation of the postoperative pain Mr. Morton is likely to experience. Also, throughout the case Dr. Long had been monitoring the degree of neuromuscular blockade with a nerve stimulator, adding small doses of vecuronium as needed to maintain paralysis. As the operation nears its conclusion, he allows the paralysis to begin to wear off without adding additional vecuronium.

STEP 8: EMERGENCE FROM ANESTHESIA

As the surgeon finishes the operation the anesthesiologist must plan for the emergence from general anesthesia that will transform the patient from the comatose and unresponsive to the awake and alert. Modern anesthetic drugs have recovery profiles that allow the anesthesiologist to awaken the anesthetized patient quickly, but still one must be careful to assure a smooth and safe transition. The usual emergence sequence includes the following:

1. Reversal of any residual neuromuscular blockade so that the patient will have full muscle strength after awakening.

2. Discontinuation of the inhaled anesthetics and administration of 100% oxygen. At this point the patient can be allowed to breath spontaneously (if not already doing so), or breathing can be continued using the ventilator. Once the inhaled anesthetic concentration is cut to zero, virtually all of the inhaled agents will be eliminated by ventilation alone. If the anesthetic had been delivered by mask or LMA, the patient will usually awaken gradually and will soon respond to commands. However, if an ETT was used the patient will often start to cough and "buck" because of irritation from the tube.

3. Extubation of the trachea (if applicable). Removal of the ETT should be delayed until the patient follows commands. (Laryngospasm can occur if he or she is extubated too early.) The anesthesiologist then suctions the oropharynx and removes the ETT. This is a critical time, as one must assure that the airway stays patent and that the patient's breathing is spontaneous and adequate.

4. Monitoring of vital signs, especially oxygen saturation, until after extubation.

5. Continued oxygen administration by simple face mask after extubation and during transfer to the PACU.

As the surgeon begins to close the surgical incision, Dr. Long gives a combination of neostigmine and glycopyrrolate to reverse any residual effects of the vecuronium. He has already allowed Mr. Morton to start breathing spontaneously, even though he remains deeply anesthetized. While the surgeon puts on the surgical dressing Dr. Long turns off the desflurane and nitrous oxide and increases the oxygen flow to 8 L/min, assuring an inspired anesthetic concentration of zero within a few seconds. After a few minutes the alveolar concentrations of desflurane and nitrous oxide have fallen to very low levels. Mr. Morton coughs briefly and then opens his eyes and squeezes Dr. Long's hand on command. After suctioning Mr. Morton's oropharynx, Dr. Long removes the ETT and gives him oxygen to breathe by face mask. Mr. Morton is breathing deeply and his oxygen saturation is 100%. He coughs and clears his throat when told to do so and then moves himself over to the stretcher. Dr. Long places a plastic face mask on Mr. Morton's face and transports him to the PACU.

STEP 9: RECOVERY FROM ANESTHESIA

After surgery and the emergence from anesthesia patients must be observed for a period of time in the PACU. After leaving the operating room, patients are admitted to the PACU where nurses with specialized training in the problems peculiar to the postsurgical patient manage most of their care. Anesthesiologists, however, continue their responsibility for the care of the patients, making themselves readily available for consultations, emergencies, and final discharge from the unit. The most common issues addressed by the PACU staff include the following:

1. Pain management.
2. Management of nausea.
3. Management of hypoxemia, or hypoventilation.
4. Management of deviations of vital signs (e.g., hypertension, hypotension, tachyarrhythmias, and bradyarrhythmias.
5. Transition of care to the home environment (if ambulatory) or the postsurgical floor (if nonambulatory).

Mr. Morton appears awake and alert in the PACU. His vital signs are all within his normal range, but he is complaining of some pain. The nurse gives him 25 µg of fentanyl intravenously, which relieves his pain. After an hour he takes an oral analgesic and moves himself to a chair. His pain seems to be under control now, even when he ambulates. The nurse removes his intravenous catheter, gives him instructions about home care, and he leaves the PACU accompanied by a family member. His total time in the hospital, from arrival until discharge, has been 8 hours.

SUMMARY

This chapter has outlined the steps involved during the administration of a simple general anesthetic. This should provide the student with a framework for a more in-depth look at general anesthetic management covered in other chapters of the handbook.

CHAPTER 3

Pharmacology and Delivery of Inhalation Anesthetics

Randall S. Glidden, MD

Ever since the days when William T.G. Morton and Crawford Long anesthetized their patients with ether, and Horace Wells used nitrous oxide for pulling teeth, anesthesiologists have depended on inhaled anesthetics to provide general anesthesia for surgical procedures. Because of their safety, efficacy, and relatively low cost, inhaled anesthetic agents constitute at least some portion of nearly all general anesthetics administered today. Although the use of ether ceased after the introduction of the halogenated volatile anesthetics in the latter half of the twentieth century, nitrous oxide is still a major component of most modern-day general anesthetics. This chapter discusses the basic principles of the use of these agents.

INHALED ANESTHETICS: TWO GROUPS

We can divide inhaled anesthetics into two groups: the volatile (or potent) anesthetics, and nitrous oxide. The volatile anesthetics (isoflurane, desflurane, and sevoflurane) are the descendants of ether. (Halothane, enflurane, and methoxyflurane are rarely used anymore.) The volatile anesthetics are liquids at room temperature, have a high vapor pressure (high volatility) and a strong ethereal odor, and can effectively anesthetize a patient when inhaled in concentrations of as little as 5% or less. Nitrous oxide, on the other hand, is an odorless gas at room temperature, is stored as a liquid in a pressurized tank, and is only a weak anesthetic, requiring high concentrations to be effective. Despite its lack of potency, nitrous oxide is much less expensive than the volatile agents, so the two are usually used in combination to reduce cost.

Because it is the inhaled route of administration that sets these agents apart from most other drugs used today, we will examine first the methods used to deliver inhaled anesthetics to the patient, how they reach the brain, and finally how they leave the body, before discussing the pharmacodynamics of the drugs themselves.

DELIVERY OF ANESTHETIC GASES: THE ANESTHESIA MACHINE AND BREATHING CIRCUIT

We all have images of the old-time country doctor anesthetizing a patient on the kitchen table using an ether-saturated cloth. Although the modern anesthesia machine is far more sophisticated than the ether-soaked cloth, it is based on similar physical principles (Fig. 3-1). Although complicated at first glance, the anesthesia machine is nothing more than a device designed to mix precise amounts of oxygen, nitrous oxide, and volatile anesthetic vapors and then deliver these gases to the patient's lungs via the anesthesia breathing circuit.

Both oxygen and nitrous oxide are supplied to the anesthesia machine via color-coded hoses (green for oxygen, blue for nitrous oxide) connected to gas outlets on the wall of the operating room, which are in turn connected to large tanks stored elsewhere in the hospital. The fittings on the hoses differ for each of the gases so that the oxygen hose cannot be attached to the nitrous oxide outlet and vice versa. As a backup to the wall gas supplies, small cylinders of oxygen and nitrous oxide are attached to the back of the anesthesia machine and can be used in the unlikely failure of the hospital supply.

Dials and flowmeters on the front of the anesthesia machine allow the anesthesiologist to regulate the flows of oxygen and nitrous oxide that will be delivered to the patient. (In addition to oxygen and nitrous oxide, most anesthesia machines are capable of delivering air to the anesthesia gas mixture if desired.) The oxygen–nitrous oxide mixture flows through a vaporizer, which adds volatile anesthetic to these gases.

The anesthesia vaporizer is the direct descendant of the ether-soaked cloth, and consists of a metal container that serves as a storage and vapor chamber for the agent, and a calibrated dial that diverts a portion of the gas mixture into the vaporizer. Because volatile anesthetics (ether included) are chemicals with high vapor pressures, they readily change from a liquid to a vapor when exposed to air at ambient temperature and pressure. For example, isoflurane has a vapor pressure of 239 mm Hg, or about one-third an atmosphere. This means that when a mixture of oxygen and nitrous oxide equilibrates with liquid isoflurane in the vaporizer chamber, isoflurane vapor will occupy approximately 33% of the resulting gas volume. Because the effective anesthetic concentration of isoflurane is approximately 1% by volume, only a small amount of the gas in the vaporizer chamber needs to be added to the oxygen-nitrous oxide mixture going to the patient to be in the anesthetic range. The calibrated dial on the vaporizer accomplishes this task by diverting a small amount of the gas mixture through the vaporizer, thus adding the required amount of volatile agent to the gases as they exit the machine and enter the anesthesia breathing circuit.

Because volatile anesthetics have different vapor pressures, specific vaporizers are used for each agent. The basic design of each is similar with the exception of the desflurane vaporizer. Because desflurane has a vapor pressure that is close to 1 atm (i.e., its boiling point is just above room temperature!), its vaporizer consists of an electronically controlled heated chamber in which the vapor is stored under pressure and then combined directly with the anesthesia gas mixture.

After the volatile agent is added to the oxygen and nitrous oxide mixture, the gases pass via a hose into the breathing circuit (also called the anesthesia circle system). As shown in the figure, gases passing into the

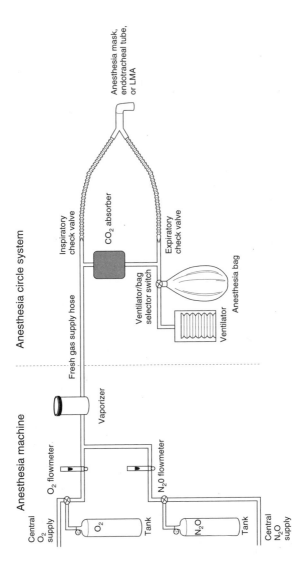

FIGURE 3-1. Anesthesia machine and breathing circuit. Note that for simplicity, the "pop-off" valve from the ventilator and anesthesia bag to the gas-scavenger system is not shown. LMA, laryngeal mask airway.

circuit flow through a one-way check valve, which opens on the patient's inspiration and closes on expiration, and then flow through the inspiratory limb of the circuit to a Y-connector. The Y-connector attaches to an anesthesia mask, a laryngeal mask airway, or an endotracheal tube.

When the patient inspires the anesthesia gases, a small amount of the nitrous oxide, oxygen, and volatile agent are taken up by the patient's pulmonary circulation and removed from the gas mixture (see "Pharmacokinetics I: Wash-in, Uptake, and Distribution of Anesthetic Gases"). After exhalation the remaining gases present in the lungs pass through the circuit's expiratory limb to another one-way check valve (opens on expiration, closes on inspiration) and enter either an anesthesia bag or a ventilator (controlled by a lever).

The anesthesia bag and the ventilator act as gas reservoirs during the respiratory cycle and also allow the anesthesiologist to apply positive pressure to the circuit if desired. Pressure relief valves attached at the anesthesia bag and at the ventilator remove excess gases from the breathing circuit by suctioning them into the hospital's vacuum system (and ultimately returning them to the outside atmosphere). Next the gases pass through a canister containing either Baralyme or Sodasorb, substances that absorb all of the expired carbon dioxide (CO_2). Gases exiting the CO_2 absorber then reenter the inspiratory limb of the breathing circuit where fresh gases from the anesthesia machine are added, and the cycle continues with the next inspiration.

Because the circle system removes all of the exhaled CO_2 from the expired gases, the patient can safely rebreathe a portion of those gases. And because the patient removes only a small quantity of the inspired volatile anesthetic and nitrous oxide from the inspired gases, the anesthesiologist can effectively recycle much of those exhaled gases by having the patient rebreathe them. In fact, by adding very low flows of fresh gases to the breathing circuit (e.g., less than 1 L/min), the patient can rebreathe up to 90% to 95% of the expired gases, thus improving the economy of the anesthetic.

By contrast, if the anesthesiologist uses high fresh gas flows, a greater proportion of fresh gas will enter the circuit and the amount of expired gases rebreathed will decrease to negligible amounts. High fresh gas flows will also cause any changes made with vaporizer settings to be reflected in a rapid change in the inspired gas concentration in the breathing circuit. This is especially important during induction and emergence when we usually quickly increase or decrease, respectively, the anesthetic gases in the patient's lungs.

PHARMACOKINETICS I: WASH-IN, UPTAKE, AND DISTRIBUTION OF ANESTHETIC GASES

Once an anesthetic gas enters a patient's lungs during inspiration, it must first mix with and reach equilibrium with the gas already present in the lungs, a process referred to as "anesthetic wash-in." As this equilibration occurs, anesthetic gases that have entered the alveoli will enter the pulmonary circulation, and then travel to the sites of action in the central nervous system (CNS), where they will exert an anesthetic effect. This second step is referred to as uptake and distribution and is key to understanding how the inhaled anesthetics reach effective levels in the CNS.

Wash-in occurs as anesthetic gases enter first the patient's upper airway and then their lungs. A certain number of breaths are required for the concentration of these gases to come into equilibrium with the gas already present in the functional residual capacity (FRC) of the patient's lungs. Because the FRC usually contains approximately 2 L of air, several breaths are necessary for the anesthetic gases to wash into the FRC and reach a concentration approaching that at which they were inhaled at the upper airway. Using relatively large tidal volumes with a rapid respiratory rate or using high inspired anesthetic gas concentrations, or both, can shorten the wash-in process.

The concept of uptake and distribution is somewhat more complicated. When a patient inhales oxygen of a given concentration, it will equilibrate with the blood passing through the alveoli of the lungs. Once in the alveoli, oxygen exerts a force directly related to its inhaled partial pressure (a function of concentration and barometric pressure) that causes it to move into the blood in the alveolar capillaries. In a similar fashion, an inhaled anesthetic gas exerts a driving force related to its partial pressure that will cause the gas to enter and gradually reach equilibrium with the pulmonary venous blood.

For example, if a patient inhales isoflurane, an amount proportional to the alveolar partial pressure will cross the alveolar membrane and enter the pulmonary venous circulation. Isoflurane will then travel in the systemic arterial blood to the rest of the body, where some of it will leave the circulation and enter the body tissues according to its solubility. The blood will return to the lungs containing somewhat less isoflurane than when it left the lungs initially; however, more isoflurane will pass from the alveoli into the pulmonary venous blood, resulting in a net increase. On each transit through the lungs and the systemic circulation, the blood concentration of isoflurane will gradually increase until it is nearly equal to the inspired concentration entering the patient's upper airway.

Solubility of an anesthetic agent in the blood and tissues of the body (usually expressed as "partition coefficient") affects the speed with which equilibration with the inspired concentration occurs. Inhaled anesthetics with low tissue solubility (e.g., desflurane, sevoflurane, and nitrous oxide) will reach equilibrium more quickly than inhaled anesthetics with higher tissue solubility (e.g., isoflurane). Because they are less soluble in the tissues, less anesthetic leaves the systemic circulation after passing through the body. More agent, therefore, remains in the venous blood as it returns to the lungs. Because more anesthetic remains in the blood returning to the lungs, less anesthetic needs to be added on the next pass through the lungs to raise the concentration closer to the inspired concentration. In this way desflurane and sevoflurane reach equilibrium with the inspired gas concentration more quickly than isoflurane, making it faster to induce anesthesia with these agents.

The anesthesiologist can observe this equilibrium effect between the inspired gas and the blood by using an anesthetic gas monitor. These monitors display the inspired concentration (or fraction inspired, FI) and the end-tidal concentration (fraction end-tidal, FET) of the commonly used anesthetic agents. The end-tidal concentration (the alveolar concentration at the end of a tidal volume breath) is in equilibrium with the blood arriving to the alveoli from the pulmonary artery and is, therefore, a reflection of the anesthetic gas concentration in the systemic blood. Because anesthetic gas in the systemic circulation is in equilibrium with the brain, the anesthesiologist uses the end-tidal concentration as an estimate of the brain concentration.

In summary, the patient inhales an anesthetic gas, and the gas washes into the FRC and alveoli. The alveolar gas enters the pulmonary circulation, travels through the body, and returns to the lungs partially depleted of anesthetic (depending on the solubility of the agent). The cycle repeats, gradually increasing the amount of anesthetic in the pulmonary circulation until the anesthetic concentration in the blood returning to the lungs, which is also the concentration to which the brain is exposed, approaches the inspired concentration.

PHARMACOKINETICS II: ELIMINATION AND EMERGENCE

Virtually all of the elimination of the modern inhaled anesthetics is by ventilation. Once the anesthesiologist shuts off the anesthetic gases coming from the anesthesia machine, the patient simply breathes out the gases that have accumulated in the body. In some ways this is the reverse of uptake and distribution because now anesthetic gases are moving from the patient's body, through the pulmonary circulation, into the lungs, and finally out into the anesthesia circuit. During this emergence phase the anesthesiologist will increase the flow of oxygen entering the breathing circuit so that little (if any) of the patient's expired gas is rebreathed. This assures that the patient will not inhale any of the expired anesthetic agents and delay emergence. The speed of emergence depends somewhat on how quickly the anesthetic gases leave the patient's body. Inhaled agents of low solubility will typically exit the body faster than those of higher solubility, because the tissues will have taken up less drug during the course of the anesthetic. Thus patients wake up faster after being anesthetized with the less soluble agents desflurane and sevoflurane than with the more soluble isoflurane.

PHARMACODYNAMICS: MINIMAL ALVEOLAR CONCENTRATION AND SYSTEMIC EFFECTS

Potency

Inhaled anesthetics exert most of their effects on the brain. As noted above, once at equilibrium the anesthetic end-tidal (alveolar) concentration is a good approximation of the brain concentration. We can compare the potencies of the various inhaled anesthetics by using the concept of minimal alveolar concentration (MAC), defined as the alveolar concentration at equilibrium necessary to prevent movement after a surgical stimulus in 50% of the patients. (This is analogous to an "effective dose 50" [ED_{50}], i.e., the dose effective in 50% of the population.) For example, the MAC for isoflurane is approximately 1.3%, whereas the MAC for desflurane is approximately 6%. Isoflurane, therefore, is approximately four times more potent than desflurane. By contrast, nitrous oxide has a MAC of 104%, rendering it virtually useless as an anesthetic if used by itself (Table 3-1).

CNS Actions

Inhaled anesthetics act in the CNS by altering neuronal activity and by decreasing transfer of sensory information. Sites of action probably include both supraspinal areas that produce loss of consciousness and amnesia and spinal areas that lead to decreased reflex movement to noxious stimuli. Although the exact mechanisms are unknown, nerve transmission is altered, perhaps by inhibiting excitatory impulses or by enhancing inhibitory impulses. We know that at the physiochemical level anesthetic potency correlates with lipid solubility—the more lipid-soluble the agent, the more potent it is (the Meyer-Overton rule). This implies that hydrophobic (lipid-soluble) sites may exist where a critical number of anesthetic molecules must gain entry to produce anesthesia. The exact location of the sites, however, and the nature of this interaction are unknown.

In addition to the CNS actions at the cellular level, volatile anesthetics (and to a lesser degree nitrous oxide) cause mild to moderate increases in cerebral blood flow when administered at concentrations above 1 MAC. This can potentially increase cerebral blood volume and intracranial pressure in patients with head trauma or intracranial masses. However, lowering the P_{CO_2} by hyperventilating the patient minimizes this undesirable effect.

Table 3-1. Characteristics of Inhaled Anesthetics

Agent	Vapor Pressure (mm Hg)	Solubility (as blood/ gas partition coefficient)	MAC (%)	% Metabolized
Diethyl ether*	440	12.00	1.90	Negligible
Halothane*	243	2.30	0.74	25–45.0
Isoflurane	239	1.40	1.15	0.2
Desflurane	664	0.45	6.00	0.2
Sevoflurane	160	0.65	2.00	1-5.0
Nitrous oxide	39,000	0.47	104.00	Negligible

*Added for historic perspective despite limited use in clinical practice.

Pulmonary and Respiratory Actions

The volatile anesthetics as a group are all potent bronchodilators. Desflurane, however, is irritating to the mucosa of the tracheobronchial tree, especially when inhaled in high concentrations, and should be used with caution in asthmatic patients as it might actually induce bronchospasm. When administered alone (i.e., without narcotics), inhaled anesthetics increase the respiratory rate but decrease the tidal volume; thus, anesthetized patients who are breathing spontaneously will have an overall slightly decreased minute ventilation. The CO_2 response curve is flattened and shifted to the right, so patients anesthetized with inhalation agents will have a higher P_{CO_2} and a lower respiratory response to changes in CO_2 production than an awake patient would.

Cardiovascular Actions

At the usual anesthetic concentrations, volatile anesthetics have minimal cardiovascular effects in healthy people. Cardiac contractility is mildly reduced and myocardial oxygen demand is usually decreased. Patients with cardiomyopathy will have a greater decrease in contractility than healthy patients; however, patients with coronary artery disease having normal cardiac contractility may benefit from the decrease in inotropy and myocardial oxygen demand caused by these agents. Volatile agents are mild peripheral vasodilators, so they decrease the systemic vascular resistance. The net effect of all the above is usually a slight decrease in blood pressure and cardiac output, which can be more pronounced in patients with underlying cardiac disease.

Other Systemic Effects

As previously mentioned, inhaled anesthetics undergo little, if any, metabolism, being almost entirely eliminated from the body by ventilation (Table 3-1). This is not the case for the now largely abandoned drug halothane, in which more than 25% of the absorbed anesthetic is metabolized, possibly causing toxic effects. Halothane was thought to be the cause of so-called halothane hepatitis, which has led to its greatly decreased use during the last two decades.

Although not thought to be a toxic effect per se, all of the volatile agents (but not nitrous oxide) are capable of triggering the syndrome known as malignant hyperthermia (MH) in susceptible individuals (see Chapter 8). Malignant hyperthermia is a disorder of intracellular skeletal muscle calcium regulation, which leads to the production of excessive heat and CO_2 in the muscle cells after exposure to certain anesthetic drugs. These drugs (often referred to as "MH triggering agents") include all of the volatile anesthetics and the depolarizing neuromuscular blocker, succinylcholine. Signs of MH in an anesthetized patient include tachycardia, elevation in CO_2 production, and high fever. The drug dantrolene, introduced in 1972, reverses the metabolic chaos taking place in the muscle cells during an MH crises by stabilizing intracellular calcium metabolism, thus returning CO_2 and heat production back to normal. Before dantrolene the mortality rate from MH was nearly 90%, but since its use worldwide mortality has fallen to less than 10%.

Although we administer the volatile anesthetics in concentrations of only approximately 1% to 6%, we usually give nitrous oxide in a concentration of 50% to 70%. Nitrous oxide is poorly soluble in tissues, but it is more soluble than nitrogen; thus, nitrous oxide can slowly diffuse into closed, air-containing structures in the body such as the viscera, increasing their volume in proportion to the partial pressure of nitrous oxide in the inspired gas (i.e., 50% inhaled nitrous oxide can double the volume of a closed gas space.) Because of this, we often do not use nitrous oxide during abdominal operations in which distension of the bowel might get in the surgeon's way.

INHALED ANESTHETIC USE DURING GENERAL ANESTHESIA

"Balanced" Anesthesia

Most anesthesiologists administering general anesthetics today use a combination of intravenous and inhaled anesthetic drugs. Because the inhaled anesthetics have a distinctive and not entirely pleasant odor, most patients prefer an intravenous induction with either sodium thiopental or propofol (see Chapters 2 and 4) followed by the maintenance of anesthesia with inhaled anesthetics. This two-step process offers the advantage of a rapid and pleasant loss of consciousness afforded by the intravenous agents and the relatively low cost and rapid emergence produced by the inhaled anesthetics.

As mentioned earlier, we normally use a gas mixture containing both nitrous oxide (in a concentration of 50% to 70%—approximately one-half MAC) and a volatile anesthetic, combined with at least 30% oxygen. Nitrous oxide is inexpensive and has low solubility, so its combination with a volatile agent both decreases the amount of volatile agent required (thus decreasing cost) and helps speed emergence from anesthesia. In addition to intravenous induction drugs, we usually administer narcotic drugs (e.g., fentanyl and morphine) during this type of anesthesia both to reduce the amount of inhaled anesthesia needed and also to provide for pain control in the immediate recovery period (see Chapter 4).

Inhalation Induction

In some circumstances the anesthesiologist may choose to induce anesthesia by a pure inhalation method, not entirely unlike the historic ether inductions of Morton and Long. For example, small children, in whom intravenous cannulation is both painful and difficult, can often be easily anesthetized using sevoflurane inhaled by mask. The pleasant-smelling sevoflurane is usually well tolerated by the child, leading to a rapid and smooth loss of consciousness. Once anesthetized, the anesthesiologist can then insert an intravenous catheter for the remainder of the procedure. As another example, patients with masses in the mediastinum may experience total airway obstruction if positive-pressure ventilation is attempted during an intravenous anesthetic induction. This inability to ventilate may persist even after placement of an endotracheal tube. In these patients the anesthesiologist will often keep the patient breathing spontaneously throughout the entire procedure by inducing anesthesia using inhaled sevoflurane and oxygen. Because inhaled anesthetics do not decrease minute ventilation significantly, this type of induction and maintenance is safe and effective to use until the surgeon can resect the mass and, thus, relieve the potential for airway obstruction.

SUMMARY

Inhaled anesthetics and the equipment used in their administration represent major components of modern anesthesia practice. From the days of ether anesthesia, inhaled anesthetics have evolved that are safe, effective, easy to administer, and relatively inexpensive and provide rapid emergence. Delivery, uptake and distribution, and recovery are easy to monitor using anesthesia gas monitors, greatly simplifying the use of these agents in the twenty-first century. Anesthesiologists usually combine inhaled agents with intravenous drugs to produce balanced anesthesia. In certain circumstances, however, inhaled anesthetics are used alone to produce complete general anesthesia.

SUGGESTED READINGS

Longnecker DE, Miller FL. Pharmacology of inhalational anesthetics. In: Rogers MC, Tinker JH, Covino BG, Longnecker DE, eds. Principles and Practice of Anesthesiology. St. Louis: Mosby Year Book, 1993:1053–1086.

Eger EI. Uptake and distribution. In: Miller RD, ed. Anesthesia. Philadelphia: Churchill Livingstone, 2000:7–95.

Petty C. The Anesthesia Machine. New York: Churchill Livingstone, 1987.

CHAPTER 4

Pharmacology of Intravenous Anesthetics and Adjuncts

Stephen A. Cohen, MD, MBA

Nearly two centuries before Morton, Long, and Wells first anesthetized their patients with inhaled agents, intravenous (IV) anesthesia was born. In 1665, Sigasmund Elsholtz injected opium intravenously into a patient in an attempt to produce anesthesia. Although the person presumably became stuporous, little further investigation ensued until nearly 200 years later. The introduction of the short-acting drug hexobarbital in 1932 stood out because it dramatically reduced induction times compared with inhalational agents. Two years later its relative, thiopental, became the gold standard for IV induction agents, securing the role of IV anesthetics in modern practice to the present. This chapter describes the principles of their use.

ADVANTAGES, DISADVANTAGES, AND USES

The ideal anesthetic drug should block sensory, reflex, mental, and motor functions. Because no perfect single agent exists, recent efforts have aimed at combining drugs in various dosages to target all aspects of general anesthesia as required by the particular patient and for a particular procedure. Available inhalational anesthetics cannot offer this degree of selectivity, because they modulate both inhibitory and excitatory neurotransmission nonspecifically. The offspring of Elsholtz's efforts have given birth to the popularity of total intravenous anesthesia (TIVA), in which specific effects can be tuned in or out by varying specific doses of different drugs.

Because none of the IV agents alone can provide "complete" anesthesia, we must use them in combinations. Most modern anesthetic regimens use a variety of IV agents along with inhalational agents. Intravenous drugs are commonly used as premedications to relieve anxiety or to produce amnesia. We also use them during the course of surgery to provide pain relief and muscle relaxation and to decrease inhalational agent requirement, postoperative nausea and vomiting (PONV), stomach volume and acidity, secretions, coughing, and breath holding.

SEDATIVE HYPNOTICS

Most sedative hypnotics (Table 4-1) exert their effects through specific interactions with the inhibitory γ-aminobutyric acid (GABA) neurotransmitter system. Activation of this system results in increased chloride con-

Table 4-1. Intravenous Sedative and Hypnotic Pharmacodynamics

Drug	CBF	CMRO$_2$	ICP	ABP	CPP	L-EEG	H-EEG	GABA	GLU
STP	↓↓↓	↓↓↓	↓	↓	↓	S-W	BS		↓
Propofol	↓↓	↓↓	↓	↓	↓	↑ β	BS	S	↓
Etomidate	↓↓↓	↓↓↓	↓			S-W	BS		
Ketamine	↑↑	↑	↑			β,θ,δ	BS		
BDZ	↓↓	↓↓*		↓**	↓	↑ β	NBS		

Abbreviations: STP, thiopental; BDZ, benzodiazepine; CBF, cerebral blood flow; CMRO$_2$, cerebral metabolic rate of oxygen utilization; *, effect reaches a plateau; ICP, intracranial pressure; ABP, arterial blood pressure; CPP, cerebral perfusion pressure; **, in the presence of hypovolemia; L-EEG, effect on EEG at low dose; H-EEG, effect on EEG at high dose; GABA, effect on deactivation or desensitization of GABA$_A$ receptor; GLU, effect on rate of glutamate release; S-W, spike and wave; BS, burst suppression; NBS, no burst suppression; S, slowed.

ductance, hyperpolarization, and neuronal inhibition. Most IV induction agents bind to a specific site denoted GABA$_A$ to enhance these cellular actions, and some also inhibit the release of the excitatory amino acid neurotransmitter glutamate.

Barbiturates

Thiopental, thiamylal, and methohexital are the most commonly used barbiturates for anesthesia. A bolus induction dose produces rapid loss of consciousness, followed by the rapid termination of central nervous system (CNS) depressant action by redistribution away from the central compartment. After a large dose of thiopental, however, metabolism to pentobarbital can prolong CNS depressant activity for many hours. Continuous infusions of barbiturates, therefore, have little role in modern anesthesia practice because of this prolonged elimination, which depends solely on hepatic metabolism.

The usual induction doses of the barbiturates produce not only unconsciousness, but also a multitude of effects on the CNS (Table 4-1). These include a reduction in intracranial pressure (ICP) owing to a decrease in cerebral oxygen consumption. Because cerebral perfusion is preserved, thiopental offers desirable properties for inducing anesthesia in many neurosurgical operations. It may also be used during periods of regional brain ischemia such as may occur during carotid endarterectomy, cerebral aneurysm surgery, hypotension, and cardiopulmonary bypass (CPB).

Barbiturates cause both respiratory and cardiac depression. They not only depress the myocardium directly, but also compromise cardiac output primarily by impeding venous return secondary to the peripheral pooling of blood.

Propofol

Propofol acts by prolonging GABA-activated chloride-channel opening and a distinct receptor-mediated tonic chloride current. Similar to thiopental, redistribution away from the central compartment after a bolus dose accounts for the rapid termination of action of propofol. Unlike thiopental, emergence occurs rapidly even after long periods of continuous infusion because of rapid clearance from the central compartment by hepatic metabolism. Table 4-1 summarizes the other CNS actions of propofol. For many neurosurgical procedures, TIVA with propofol and narcotics provides the most desirable conditions by lowering ICP and providing a slack brain.

In normal adults, the induction dose of propofol is 1.5 to 2.5 mg/kg. Continuous infusions of 100 to 200 μg/kg per minute maintain unconsciousness. Because of a larger central volume of distribution in children and a smaller one in the elderly, these dosages must be adjusted upward or downward, respectively.

Propofol affects respiratory function by initially decreasing tidal volume and increasing respiratory rate. The response to increased $Paco_2$ and decreased Pao_2 is blunted, and at higher doses apnea occurs. Propofol directly depresses the myocardium and decreases systemic vascular resistance secondary to both arterial and venous vasodilation, which is quantitatively greater than that produced by thiopental. Propofol not only produces little nausea and vomiting, it actually appears to possess antiemetic activity.

Etomidate

Etomidate works by augmenting the GABA-activated chloride conductance at the $GABA_A$ receptor complex, and, at higher concentrations, directly eliciting chloride currents. Its usefulness results from its minimal depression of cardiovascular and pulmonary function. It is ideal for inducing anesthesia in patients with a compromised cardiovascular system, cerebrovascular disease, or hemodynamic instability. Opioids are commonly used in these instances to blunt the response to laryngoscopy.

The induction dose of etomidate, 0.2 to 0.4 mg/kg, commonly causes pain on injection and produces myoclonic movements. Emergence from etomidate is rapid even after continuous infusion. Use of the drug for anesthesia maintenance has fallen out of favor, however, because of its purported suppression of cortisol synthesis. When used with narcotics, etomidate produces a particularly high incidence of postoperative nausea and vomiting. The actions of etomidate on the CNS and cerebrovascular system are summarized in Table 4-1. Although it can provoke myoclonic activity, at high doses it behaves as a prominent anticonvulsant.

Ketamine

Ketamine exerts its anesthetic properties through antagonism of the excitatory N-methyl-D-aspartate receptor channel complex, presumably by binding to the open channel. Ketamine, too, minimally depresses the cardiorespiratory system.

The usual IV induction dose of ketamine, 1 to 2 mg/kg, produces a dissociative anesthetic state of not only unconsciousness and amnesia but also analgesia, in which the thalamocortical and limbic systems become functionally segregated. Emergence occurs 10 to 20 minutes later, but profound disorientation may last for 1.5 hours after a single dose or considerably longer after continuous infusion.

Soon after consciousness returns, ketamine commonly produces hallucinations, nightmares, and impaired cognition and short-term memory. It affects cerebrovascular hemodynamics differently from other agents discussed thus far (Table 4-1), thereby making it generally unsuitable for use in patients with increased ICP. The bronchodilator action of ketamine makes it desirable for use in patients with bronchospastic disease, but its sialogogic action increases the likelihood of laryngospasm during light anesthesia. Its direct stimulation of the sympathetic nervous system (SNS) causes an increase in heart rate and blood pressure. The resulting increased myocardial oxygen consumption renders ketamine a poor choice for patients with coronary artery disease. However, it also possesses a direct myocardial depressant action (usually offset by the indirect SNS stimulation), which may result in hypotension in chronically ill persons whose catecholamines have been depleted.

Benzodiazepines

Benzodiazepines (BDZs) are another important class of sedatives. Their binding to the $GABA_A$ receptor complex increases the coupling efficiency between the receptor and chloride conductance thereby producing larger inhibitory postsynaptic currents. The anxiolytic effect progresses to one of sedation and unconsciousness with increasing BDZ receptor occupancy. The compounds also have amnestic, hypnotic, anticonvulsant, and CNS-mediated muscle relaxing actions.

The most important BDZs in anesthesia practice are midazolam, diazepam, and lorazepam. They are usually used as a premedication to provide anxiolysis and sedation before general anesthesia or during local or regional anesthesia. Midazolam, in induction doses of 0.1 to 0.2 mg/kg and infusion rates of 0.25 to 1 μg/kg per minute, can render unconsciousness; however, prolonged recovery time argues against this practice.

BDZ administration produces respiratory, cardiovascular, and upper airway reflex depression. In healthy patients, these effects are generally not clinically relevant, but may become significant if other depressants such as narcotics are also given. In the presence of hypovolemia, the decrease in preload and afterload caused by BDZs can cause substantial hypotension.

The unique high-affinity competitive antagonist of BDZs, flumazenil, reverses the sedative action of these compounds. Because the biologic half-life of flumazenil is only approximately 1 hour, resedation may occur unless given in subsequent doses or by continuous infusion. Flumazenil must be used cautiously because its antagonism of ventilatory depression is incomplete, and it can produce acute elevation of ICP in patients with a head injury by a yet undetermined mechanism.

ANALGESICS

Narcotics

Since ancient times people have used opium for the treatment of pain. It is a natural extract of the poppy (*Papaver somniferum*) that contains more than 20 alkaloids including morphine and codeine, the former being the first pure opioid used in medicine. Although morphine's properties were well studied throughout the nineteenth century, its use in anesthesia awaited the development of neuromuscular blocking drugs and the development of mechanical ventilation.

In the late 1950s, so-called opioid anesthesia using morphine for cardiac surgery blossomed. Fentanyl, a synthetic narcotic introduced in 1960, had much greater potency and margin of safety and therefore often supplanted morphine during surgery. The other fentanyl derivatives, sufentanil and alfentanil, were developed in the mid-1970s in an attempt to maximize specific properties such as potency, rapidity of onset, and duration of action. In 1996, remifentanil, a narcotic with an ultrashort duration of action because of the rapid hydrolysis of its ester side chain, gained US Food and Drug Administration (FDA) approval.

Much has been learned about opioid action in the last 30 years. In 1973 high-affinity opioid binding sites in mammalian brain tissue were discovered. Three subtypes of sites were identified based on the ability of the three agonists morphine, ketocyclazocine, and DADLE [(D-Ala, D-Leu]enkephalin) to compete for binding. The receptors so described were called mu (μ), kappa (κ), and delta (δ), respectively. The original description of multiple receptors has been substantially broadened. Currently, strong evidence exists for three subtypes of μ—μ_1, μ_2, and μ_3; two subtypes of δ—δ_1, δ_2; and three subtypes of κ—κ_1, κ_2, and κ_3. All can mediate analgesia but display other discrete pharmacologic functions as well.

The different receptor types show not only different ligand binding, but also different distributions and function. Thus, physiologic opioid responses generally result from the action of the drug at multiple sites. Effects of opioids include analgesia, miosis, bradycardia, sedation, and hypothermia. The most thoroughly studied action is analgesia for which it has been shown that opioids inhibit neurotransmitter release from dorsal root ganglion cells. Naturally occurring endogenous peptides such as enkephalins, endorphins, and dynorphins show binding specificity for the receptor subtypes. The most clinically useful narcotics, morphine and fentanyl, display high, but not total, μ specificity.

Opioid receptors are coupled to guanine nucleotide binding proteins (G proteins). These complexes not only stimulate the second messenger adenylate cyclase system, but also appear to mediate ionic current flows, which result in neuronal hyperpolarization.

Physicochemical properties determine the ability of opioids to cross the blood-brain barrier and interact with their receptors. Generally speaking, greater lipid solubility and nonionized fraction results in greater membrane permeability. Binding to plasma proteins retards transport across the blood-brain barrier.

Morphine represents the gold standard for μ agonists against which all others are compared. It acts at several levels in the CNS synergistically to produce analgesia. For example, in the spinal cord its action is mediated by μ_2 receptors, whereas in supraspinal centers it affects mostly μ_1 receptors. Primary afferent neurons may also possess opioid receptors, which when activated can produce analgesia.

Other CNS effects include drowsiness, cognitive impairment, mood alteration, nausea, inhibition of corticotropin-releasing factor and antidiuretic hormone release, and sleep disturbances.

Morphine and other opioids depress breathing principally by impairing the medullary response to CO_2, which ultimately leads to apnea. The medullary cough center is depressed, too, which results in attenuation of the cough reflex. In large doses, morphine can produce abdominal muscle and chest wall rigidity, which seems to be the result of central μ activation. Morphine directly stimulates the chemoreceptor trigger zone (CTZ), which may produce nausea. The CTZ in turn can stimulate the vomiting center to generate emesis. All three main types of opioid receptors play roles in morphine's actions on the gastrointestinal (GI) tract. For example, GI motility and propulsion and gastric secretion are all decreased by μ receptor stimulation. Morphine produces urinary retention by stimulation of μ or δ receptors. It stimulates basophils and lung and skin mast cells to release histamine. Moderate doses of morphine have little effect on blood pressure and heart rate and rhythm in normovolemic patients. It can produce vascular dilation (probably mediated through histamine release), decrease systemic vascular resistance, and impair baroreceptor reflexes leading to orthostatic hypotension. These hemodynamic variables in patients with high sympathetic tone respond more dramatically to morphine administration. Hence, critically ill or hypovolemic patients may display exaggerated hemodynamic responses (i.e., hypotension) after even small doses of morphine. Opioids produce bradycardia but do not significantly depress myocardial contractility at usual doses.

Analgesic dosages of morphine range from 0.01 to 0.20 mg/kg. As the sole intraoperative anesthetic, doses as high as 3.0 mg/kg can be used.

Meperidine is the prototype of the phenylpiperidine class of opioids. Its analgesic potency is approximately one tenth that of morphine and appears to be mediated mostly by μ, but also by some κ and δ, receptor activation. In addition to the side effects seen with morphine, it can also produce seizures in therapeutic dosages. Meperidine possesses weak local anesthetic action, which may be responsible for its depressant effect on myocardial contractility. In general it causes greater hemodynamic instability than morphine or fentanyl.

The IV analgesic dose of meperidine varies between 0.1 and 1 mg/kg. In doses of 12.5 to 50 mg, meperidine reduces the shivering commonly seen after anesthesia, in transfusion reactions, and with fever.

Structurally similar to meperidine, the derivatives of 4-anilinopiperidine, fentanyl, sufentanil, alfentanil, and remifentanil, are the most commonly used narcotics in clinical anesthesia. Fentanyl is a strong μ agonist, which is 50 to 100 times more potent than morphine. Thus, a single IV fentanyl dose of 1.5 μg/kg 5 minutes before skin incision decreases either the inhalational agent's minimal alveolar concentration requirement or the TIVA propofol requirement by approximately two thirds.

In clinical practice, fentanyl 1.5 to 5 μg/kg is given 3 to 5 minutes before sedative-hypnotic administration to blunt the response to laryngoscopy and intubation. It is used in "balanced anesthesia," (the combination of narcotic, nitrous oxide, and neuromuscular blocker, with or without a potent inhalational agent) in boluses of 0.5 to 2.5 μg/kg every 30 to 45 minutes. Continuous infusions of 2 to 10 μg/kg per hour after a loading dose of 5 to 10 μg/kg can also be used.

For patients with significant coronary artery disease, fentanyl is sometimes used as the sole anesthetic agent. In doses of 50 to 150 μg/kg, fentanyl all but completely attenuates the stress response to surgical stimulation. This technique produces hemodynamic stability with little myocardial depression. Unconsciousness usually ensues with these high doses of fentanyl, but instances of awareness have been reported.

Sufentanil is also a μ agonist analgesic, which is 5 to 15 times as potent as fentanyl. The indications for sufentanil use are similar to those for fentanyl with dosages suitably adjusted. The greater lipid solubility of sufentanil promotes blood-brain barrier penetration, which confers a more rapid onset of action.

Alfentanil also produces analgesia by μ receptor activation but is one fourth to one tenth as potent as fentanyl. Because 90% of alfentanil exists in the nonionized form at physiologic pH, it penetrates the CNS rapidly and exerts analgesic activity within 1 minute of administration. Because its duration of action is also brief, it is useful in short surgical procedures. It can produce hypotension with the concurrent administration of other medications.

The newest opioid, remifentanil, shows specific (μ-mediated analgesia approximately 2 to 10 times as potent as fentanyl with virtually undetectable δ and κ activity. It possesses a rapid onset and extremely short duration of action because of termination by blood and tissue esterases so that even after prolonged administration it does not accumulate. It is usually administered as a continuous infusion at a rate of 0.05 to 0.5 (μg/kg per minute.

Nonsteroidal Anti-inflammatory Drugs

Nonsteroidal anti-inflammatory drugs (NSAIDs) are playing an increasingly important role in surgical pain management. They work by inhibiting cyclooxygenase, which promotes the synthesis of prostaglandins (PGs) and other autacoids, and by direct action on sensory neurons.

Cyclooxygenase catalyzes the conversion of arachidonic acid to the cyclic endoperoxides PGG_2 and PGH_2, which are further degraded depending on the tissue enzymes present. Two forms of the cyclooxygenase enzyme exist: cyclooxygenase-1 (COX-1) and cyclooxygenase-2 (COX-2). The former resides in most cells including those of blood vessel endothelium, platelets, stomach mucosa, and kidney collecting tubules. Inflammation products such as cytokines and growth factors induce the latter enzyme.

NSAIDs can produce significant side effects such as GI ulceration, inhibition of thromboxane synthesis and platelet aggregation, diminished uterine motility inhibition, renal dysfunction, and hypersensitivity reactions. Most NSAIDs are administered orally and inhibit COX-1 and COX-2 nondiscriminantly. Recently, selective COX-2 inhibitors (e.g., rofecoxib, celecoxib) have been developed in an effort to diminish these adverse reactions.

At present, one nonspecific COX inhibitor IV agent, ketorolac, is used in clinical anesthesia. Parecoxib, an IV selective COX-2 inhibitor, is in phase III clinical trials and is still awaiting final FDA approval (May 2002).

NEUROMUSCULAR BLOCKING DRUGS

Therapeutic uses of neuromuscular blocking drugs include facilitating tracheal intubation and certain types of surgery when relaxation of skeletal muscle is desirable. They are also used when light anesthesia is administered to a patient who would not tolerate the cardiorespiratory depressant effects of deeper anesthesia, or when a more rapid awakening and shortened recovery period are sought.

We typically monitor neuromuscular blockade by electrically stimulating a suitable peripheral nerve and assessing the muscle twitch response. This permits us to obtain reliable operating conditions and assure that after the procedure recovery is adequate to sustain respiratory function. Either "train-of-four" or "double-burst" patterns of stimuli are commonly used. In either, the percentage of blocked acetylcholine receptors (AChR) can be estimated from the number of twitches seen and the ratio of the last to the first twitch height in response to a series of electrical shocks applied to the innervating nerve.

Depolarizing Blocking Drug

Neuromuscular blockers can be classified depending on whether or not they depolarize the postsynaptic membrane of the neuromuscular junction. The only depolarizing blocking drug used clinically in the United States is succinylcholine (SCh), which exhibits biphasic action. In phase I it activates AChRs, and cation conductivity markedly increases, which results in muscle depolarization. During prolonged administration, the continued presence of SCh at the motor endplate desensitizes the AChRs there, which cease to respond to nerve impulses. The membrane remains depolarized, and after a time, the block characteristics change to a so-called phase II type. In this phase, neuromuscular transmission is blocked at the perijunctional muscle membrane at which the voltage-dependent sodium channels have become inactivated because of the sustained depolarization.

SCh doses of 1 mg/kg produce conditions suitable for endotracheal intubation in approximately 1 minute. Important common side effects of SCh administration include fasciculations, myalgias, increased intraocular pressure, increased intracranial pressure, and hyperkalemia. In the rare patient, SCh can trigger malignant hyperthermia (see Chapters 3 and 8), and prolonged paralysis can occur (3 to 6 hours) in patients with abnormal or absent plasma cholinesterase.

Nondepolarizing Blocking Drugs

Unlike SCh, nondepolarizing blockers bind competitively to the AChR. Hence, their blockade can be reversed by using the anticholinesterase drugs neostigmine and edrophonium, which increase the amount of acetylcholine (ACh) present at the neuromuscular junction. Anticholinergic agents such as glycopyrrolate or atropine must be administered contemporaneously to prevent profound cardiovascular vagal effects produced by increased levels of ACh at muscarinic receptors.

Nondepolarizing agents can be divided into two classes: the benzylisoquinolines and the ammonio steroids. Many such compounds have been developed during the last 60 years, but fewer than 10 are commonly used in clinical practice today. Table 4-2 shows their properties. A specific agent may be selected for particular characteristics such as its onset and duration of action or side effects.

Clinically significant interactions between neuromuscular blockers and other drugs exist. For example, potentiation occurs with the inhalational agents, lidocaine, antibiotics such as neomycin, streptomycin, gentamicin, and clindamycin, and acute phenytoin therapy. Chronic anticonvulsant administration confers resistance to many nondepolarizing agents, and acute administration enhances their block. A pharmacokinetic explanation (i.e., enhanced liver enzyme-dependent degradation) probably accounts for the former, whereas a pharmacodynamic reason likely explains the latter.

ANTIEMETICS

Patients rate nausea and vomiting among the most undesired side effects after general anesthesia. Hence, preventing or treating these symptoms is an integral part of the practice of anesthesiology. The emetic response is complex, and preventing it requires some understanding of the process. The vomiting center in the medulla receives afferents from the CTZ in the area

Table 4-2. Properties of Commonly Used Neuromuscular Blockers

Drug	Structure	Onset (min)	Duration (min)	Potency ED$_{95}$ (μg/kg)	T$_{90}$ (min)	T$_{1/2\beta}$ (min)	Mode of Elimination
Succinylcholine	DE	0.75–1.5	6–8	25			H
Rocuronium	AS	1–2	30–40	300	20	130	L, R
Mivacurium	B	2–4	12–18	80–150	20	1.8	H
Atracurium	B	2–4	30–40	200	20–25	20	Hf, H
Vecuronium	AS	2–4	30–40	80	20	110	L, R
d-Tubocurarine	CB	4–6	80–120	500	70–90	90–350	R, LC
Pancuronium	AS	4–6	120–180	60	60	100–130	R, L, LC
Pipecuronium	AS	2–4	80–100	30–48	60	120–150	R
Cisatracurium	B	2–4	30–40	50	20–25	20	Hf, H

Abbreviations: DE, dicholine ester; B, benzylisoquinoline; CB, cyclic benzylisoquinoline; AS, ammonio steroid; T$_{90}$, time to 90% recovery after an ED$_{95}$; T$_{1/2\beta}$, elimination half-life; H, hydrolysis by plasma cholinesterases; Hf, Hofman degradation; L, liver metabolism; LC, liver clearance; R, renal elimination; LC, liver clearance.

postrema of the medulla, vestibular apparatus, higher brainstem and cortical structures, pharynx, GI tract, and visual center. The CTZ contains dopamine (D2), serotonin (5-HT$_3$), histamine (H$_1$), and muscarinic (M) receptors. Because of a poorly developed blood-brain barrier in the area postrema, circulating substances can stimulate the CTZ directly.

Antiemetics fall into five main classes, which are antagonists of 5-HT$_3$, D2, H$_1$, and M receptors, and other compounds acting by yet unknown mechanisms. The 5-HT$_3$ antagonists ondansetron, granisetron, and dolasetron, along with the D2 antagonist metoclopramide, are considered among the most effective antiemetics. Other D2 antagonists such as the phenothiazines (e.g., prochlorperazine) provide antiemetic effect for mild-to-moderate nausea. The H$_1$ antagonists such as diphenhydramine or antimuscarinics such as scopolamine are somewhat less effective and generally produce considerable sedation. Corticosteroids, whose mechanism of action is unknown, have come into greater use recently.

SUMMARY

IV anesthetics not only complement inhaled agents but also can be used alone to attain the most desirable characteristics of a general anesthetic. Modern IV agents have been developed that are efficacious and safe. They provide the means to block reliably and reversibly sensory, reflex, mental, and motor functions.

SUGGESTED READINGS

Chebib M, Johnston GAR. GABA-activated ligand gated ion channels: medicinal chemistry and molecular biology. J Med Chem 2000;43:142–1447.

Cherubini E, Conti F. Generating diversity at GABAergic synapses. Trends Neurosci. 2001;24:155-162.

Minami M, Satoh M. Molecular biology of the opioid receptors: structures, functions and distributions. Neurosci Res 1995;23:121–145.

Jordan BA, Cvejic S, Devi LA. Opioids and their complicated receptor complexes. Neuropsychopharmacology 2000;23(Suppl):S5– S18.

CHAPTER 5

Pharmacology of Local Anesthetics and Regional Anesthesia

Christopher Quartararo, MD

INTRODUCTION

Although much of the time spent in an anesthesia rotation deals with patients under general anesthesia, often it is a regional anesthetic that leaves the strongest impression on a student. Upper or lower extremity surgery under peripheral nerve block is fascinating, but a colon resection or a cesarean section in an awake patient or the pain relief provided by an epidural catheter is almost magical.

First we should define local and regional anesthesia. In local anesthesia a local anesthetic drug is injected directly into the site of the surgical incision, whereas in regional anesthesia the anesthetic is injected around the nerve that supplies the operative field. For example, if you are going to suture a hand laceration under local anesthesia, the anesthetic is injected directly into the skin at the site of the laceration, whereas for a regional anesthetic an injection could be made into the brachial plexus at the axilla, anesthetizing the entire arm. Patients having procedures that require a large anesthetized area are good candidates for regional anesthesia as are dental and orthopedic procedures, inasmuch as teeth and bones cannot be injected with a local anesthetic.

HISTORY

Although regional anesthesia as we know it today is a relatively recent discovery, the rendering of body parts numb by physical means is an ancient procedure. Ice can be used to quell the pain of an injury or even render it anesthetic, and ischemic anesthesia can be accomplished by compression of the artery that supplies an extremity.

Before what we now call regional anesthesia could be practiced, three things were needed: first, the understanding that sensation and motor control are transmitted by a nervous system; second, the availability of anesthetic drugs that can reversibly disrupt the transmission of nerve impulses; and third, a method for delivering these drugs to the required area. With the invention of the glass syringe and hollow needle in the 1850s and discovery of cocaine in 1884, the stage was set for the development of regional anesthesia. General anesthesia was approximately 40 years old by then, and, although it was a great advance, its dangers had become clear. However, the hopes for a safe and effective alternative to general anesthesia were only realized once the highly toxic cocaine was replaced by procaine (Novocaine) in 1904, followed by the development of other synthetic local anesthetics.

MANAGEMENT OF A REGIONAL ANESTHETIC

Patient Selection

Patients are sometimes reluctant to accept a regional anesthetic as opposed to a general anesthetic. The operating room is a foreign and frightening environment for them, and they are often facing an unpleasant or even disfiguring procedure. They may have heard stories about people becoming paralyzed after a spinal anesthetic or of painful spinal taps in the emergency room. They may also be unable to believe that they could have an operation while awake and still be comfortable, or that they could stay still during the procedure. So it is understandable that many patients desire to be "put out" until the operation is over. Although no one should be pressured into accepting a regional anesthetic, once someone has been convinced to proceed, it often becomes that individual's anesthetic of choice.

On the other hand, there are patients who are frightened by the loss of control that general anesthesia imposes. These patients welcome the option of being awake for their procedure. Other people are just curious about what is happening to them and enjoy being able, for example, to watch their knee arthroscopy while it is happening. Regional anesthesia for cesarean section allows mothers to be at their baby's birth and has been proven to be safer for mother and child. It allows patients to undergo shoulder or hand surgery and go home almost immediately. Finally, by avoiding general anesthesia many patients can avoid such side effects as nausea and vomiting, sore throat, and muscle aches.

Of course not all patients are suitable for regional anesthesia. If a patient is unable to communicate with the anesthesia team (either because of language difficulties or because of some psychological problem), then assessment of the adequacy of the block or of the patient's comfort may be impossible. Infection at the injection site and coagulopathy are absolute contraindications to spinal and epidural anesthesia as these increase the risk of meningitis and hematoma. Patients who have limited cardiac output because of valvular disease or pump failure and are preload and afterload dependent are not good candidates for spinal anesthesia as it can lead to life-threatening hypotension. Patients with chronic obstructive pulmonary disease or with obesity may be intolerant of any respiratory muscle weakness induced by spinal, epidural, or interscalene blocks.

Some procedures do not lend themselves to regional techniques. Because all awake patients will shift position and occasionally cough, procedures that are intolerant to motion are better served with general anesthesia (perhaps with paralysis). Surgery around the diaphragm (which includes laparoscopy because the CO_2 insufflation is a diaphragmatic irritant) and thoracic surgery (which requires positive-pressure ventilation) are difficult if not impossible to perform under regional blockade. Surgery that requires strong traction on the viscera can be uncomfortable despite adequate somatic blockade because some visceral sensation is mediated by the vagus nerve. Procedures requiring incisions at multiple sites in different nervous distributions may prove too difficult for a regional anesthetic. Finally, extremely long procedures and those requiring awkward positioning are hard to tolerate while awake, no matter how well the surgical site is anesthetized.

Preparation

A regional anesthetic requires the same preoperative care, the same attention to details, and the same vigilance as a general anesthetic does. The central blocks (spinal and epidural) can cause major physiologic insult requiring intervention. Peripheral blocks have an incidence of systemic toxicity and can fail even in the best of hands. Even a successful block can be rendered inadequate if the surgical site must be extended outside the anesthetic area or if the duration of surgery is longer than expected. Because of this, the anesthesiologist should always be fully prepared to perform a general anesthetic if necessary.

Although not always necessary, it is often quite helpful if patients are given some sedation. They should be warned that the injection required may hurt a bit, and they should understand that they might feel some touching or other sensations during their operation. They should have a general understanding of the surgical and anesthetic procedures and have a rapport with the anesthesiologist before the anesthetic is begun.

Equipment

In addition to the equipment required for general anesthesia, regional anesthesia requires only a few syringes, some local anesthetic, and an assortment of needles. The needles used for nerve blocks are specially designed to help avoid nerve injury. They have pencil point or short beveled tips and are often difficult to pass through the skin. If a nerve stimulator is used, then an insulated needle can make positioning more accurate because the current flow is limited to the tip of the needle.

When placing a block, the workspace should have good lighting and all the necessary supplies within reach. Equipment for maintaining the airway must be at hand, including suction, a suction handle, a hand ventilator (Ambu bag) with mask, oxygen, and routine monitors (i.e., electrocardiogram, pulse oximeter, and blood pressure cuff). There should also be quick access to emergency intubation supplies and such drugs as an intravenous (IV) induction agent, succinylcholine, atropine, and something to increase blood pressure.

LOCAL ANESTHETICS

Chemically, local anesthetics consist of a hydrophilic group (usually a tertiary amine) linked to a lipophilic structure by a carbon chain, which usually contains either an ester or amide bond (Table 5-1). Thus the local anesthetics are characterized as esters or amides. The esters are hydrolyzed in the blood or liver whereas the amides are generally dealkylated in the liver.

Table 5-1. Pharmacology or Commonly Used Local Anesthetics

Drug	Type	Relative Potency (vs. Lidocaine)	Available Concentrations (%)	Maximum Dose (mg/kg)	Maximum Dose With Epi (mg/kg)	Onset Time	Duration of Action (h) Spinal/Block	Comments
Bupivacaine	Amide	4	0.25%, 0.5%, 0.75%	2.5	3	Moderate	2–4/5–18	Initial toxic effect may be sudden cardiovascular collapse
Chloroprocaine	Ester	0.5	2%, 3%	12	15	Fast	NA/0.5–1.5	Least toxic
Etidocaine	Amide	3	1%	4	5	Fast	NA/3–12	Motor blockade is greater than sensory blockade
Lidocaine	Amide	1	0.5%, 1%, 1.5% 2%, 4%, 5%	4.5	7	Fast	1–1.5/1.5–3	Most widely used, many topical preparations
Mepivacaine	Amide	1	1%, 2%, 3%	5	8	Fast	1–1.5/2–3	Similar pharmacokinetics to lidocaine
Prilocaine	Amide	1	4% (dental)	8	8	Fast	NA/1.5–3	Least toxic amide may cause methemoglobinemia
Procaine	Ester	0.5	1%, 2%, 10%	15	15	Slow	0.5–1/0.5–1.5	First synthetic local (Novocain)
Ropivacaine	Amide	3	0.25%, 0.5%, 0.75%, 1%	3	4	Moderate	2–4/5–12	May be less cardiotoxic than bupivacane
Tetracaine	Ester	4	1%	1	2	Slow	2–3/NA	Most toxic ester
Cocaine	Ester	1	1%, 4%, 10%	1	NA	NA	NA/NA	Topical only, good vasol constrictor, often used for nasal mucosa, high toxicity

Note: Maximum dosages are dependent on the location of delivery. Plasma levels vary greatly with nerve block site and between patients.
NA, not applicable.

Despite these groupings the local anesthetics are more alike than different. These drugs work by diffusing into the axon and blocking the sodium channels, thus making the axon unable to transmit impulses. Because of the tertiary amine group, these drugs are all weak bases, with a pKa (negative logarithm of the ionization constant of the acid) between 7.5 and 9.5, and are dispensed dissolved as salts of a strong acid (often hydrochloride).

The rate of onset of each drug depends on concentration, molecular weight, degree of protein binding, and degree of ionization. To enter the cell these drugs must be in the un-ionized form, whereas inside the cell the ionized form is active. Adding sodium bicarbonate to a local anesthetic solution will increase the ratio of un-ionized to ionized drug, and decrease the onset time of the block, but it will increase the risk of precipitation of the solution. Lidocaine and mepivacaine tend to have rapid onset, whereas bupivacaine and tetracaine have much slower onsets.

The duration of a block is dependent on how long the local anesthetic remains at therapeutic concentration at the site of injection. Uptake from the site is dependent on the drug's diffusion, solubility, and protein binding and on the blood flow in the area. The duration of a block is adjusted by choosing which drug to inject and can be lengthened by the addition of vasoconstrictors, such as epinephrine, which decrease blood flow. If no drug has a long enough length of action, then a catheter can be inserted at the site and multiple injections or a continuous infusion can be used. Bupivacaine and tetracaine have long durations whereas procaine, chloroprocaine, and lidocaine are shorter acting.

Systemic toxicity is related to the blood plasma level, which depends on the rate of uptake compared with the rate of clearance of a drug. Intercostal nerve blocks produce the highest blood levels because these blocks are performed over several different sites, the chest wall is well perfused, and the anesthetic is thought to spread over a reasonably large area between the ribs. Injections into the highly vascular epidural space also produce high blood levels in contrast to blocks of the feet and hands, which give lower levels. Because vasoconstrictors decrease drug uptake, they will decrease peak blood levels and allow a higher total dose of drug to be given. Clearance of local anesthetics is dependent on redistribution and metabolism. Chloroprocaine, which is rapidly cleared from the blood, gives the lowest blood levels whereas tetracaine, another ester, has a long half-life and is quite toxic.

Toxicity usually starts with sedation and progresses to excitement, unconsciousness, convulsions, respiratory depression, and finally cardiovascular collapse. The cardiotoxicity seen with bupivacaine may precede mental and respiratory symptoms, so the use of this drug deserves special care.

NEUROANATOMY

To understand and perform regional anesthesia, it is important to know the anatomy of the central and peripheral nervous systems (Fig. 5-1)The spinal canal extends from the foramen magnum to the sacral hiatus and is formed

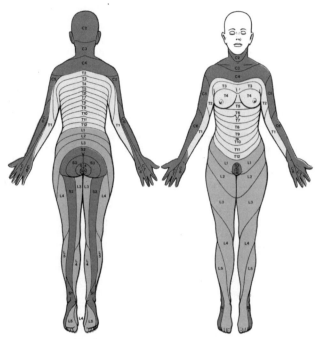

FIGURE 5-1. Dermatomal chart. The segmental areas are illustrated to emphasize the most reliable cutaneous area to test for blockade of individual spinal cord segments. (Reprinted with permission from Cousins MJ, Bridenbaugh PO. Neural Blockade in Clinical Anesthesia and Management of Pain, 3rd Ed. Baltimore: Lippincott Williams & Wilkins, 1997:312.)

by the vertebrae and their ligaments. Of note are the ligamentum flavum, the interspinous ligaments, and the supraspinous ligament, which are the dorsal ligaments of the back. The ligamenta flava are very tough paired ligaments that attach from the lower aspect of the lamina of one vertebra to the upper aspect of the next and extend from the foramina laterally to the midline, where they are usually fused. The other dorsal ligaments are in the midline, with the interspinous ligaments between the spinous processes and the supraspinous ligament dorsal to them. The tough dura mater sits within this canal. It is fused to the periostium at the foramen magnum and terminates caudally in the filum of the dura mater around the second sacral space.

Between the dura and the vertebral canal is the epidural space, which is really a potential space, containing only veins, arteries, and small amounts of fat. The more delicate arachnoid membrane is deep to the dura and separated from it by another potential space called the subdural space, which contains only a thin layer of fluid. The arachnoid gets its name from the weblike trabeculae that cross the cerebrospinal fluid (CSF)-filled subarachnoid space and attach to the pia mater, which is in turn attached to the spinal cord. The spinal cord extends the length of the vertebral canal during initial fetal development, but it does not elongate as fast as the canal does. Because of this, the spinal cord terminates at the third or fourth lumbar vertebra in the newborn, and by adulthood it extends to only the second lumbar vertebra. The nerve roots must travel caudally through the CSF from their origin at the cord to the vertebral foramina, where they exit the canal. The collection of nerve roots caudal to the terminus of the spinal cord is termed the cauda equina.

When the nerve roots leave the spinal canal the meninges (dura, arachnoid, and pia) are carried along with them and fuse with the connective tissue sheaths of the nerves. This fusion takes place outside the spinal canal, so short cuffs of dura containing CSF (which is contiguous with the main subarachnoid space) are exposed. The plexus formed from the merging and branching of the nerve roots gives rise to the peripheral nerves. Each nerve is composed of several bundles of nerve fibers held together by an epineurium, with each bundle covered by a perineurium. These bundles may branch and join inside a nerve, causing further mixing of axons from different spinal levels and of different functional classes. As the nerves pass more distally their course becomes more variable but will usually retain the same relative position to other structures such as the muscles and arteries. By using these structures as landmarks, the anesthesiologist can identify a general area where the nerves can be searched.

Nerve fibers are divided into three groups. The A fibers, which are somatic motor and sensory nerves, are large and highly myelinated and require the highest concentrations of local anesthetic to block them. The B fibers are small and slightly myelinated and innervate vascular smooth muscle. The C fibers are small and unmyelinated, are the easiest to block, and carry the sensation of pain and temperature. This is why the sensations of temperature and pain are blocked first and are more extensive than that of somatic blockade.

SPINAL (SUBARACHNOID) ANESTHESIA

Regional anesthesia is accomplished by bathing the nerves in a local anesthetic solution of sufficient concentration to render the axon nonexcitable. These nerve fibers are most exposed in the subarachnoid space. Therefore, if small amounts of local anesthetic are mixed with the CSF that bathes the nerve roots, complete block of impulses is quickly achieved. Because the spinal cord ends at the first or second lumbar vertebra, a needle can be passed into the subarachnoid space below this level without fear of hitting the cord.

The subarachnoid space is intolerant to contaminants, whether they are infectious, chemical, or physical. In any procedure in which this space is potentially entered, care must be taken to avoid contamination. The puncture site must be cleaned and prepared with a disinfectant to kill skin bacteria and viruses. Also one must avoid dragging skin cells into the spinal canal as these cells are epithelial in nature and are designed for an external surface where they can grow, die, and slough. In an enclosed space the sloughing cells will form a space-occupying lesion that can put pressure on the contents of the spinal canal. For this reason all spinal needles are constructed with a stylette to prevent skin coring. This stylette also adds stiffness to the fine-caliber needles used for this block. Finally, the injected drugs must be suitable for spinal anesthesia and be preservative free.

To place the needle in the subarachnoid space, the patient is positioned in either the lateral or sitting position with the back flexed to open the interspinous spaces. For a midline approach, the midline is identified, and local anesthetic is injected into the skin to produce an anesthetic area for the needle insertion. The spinal needle is placed fairly perpendicular to the skin and passed through the skin, subcutaneous fat, supraspinus ligament, interspinous ligament, ligamentum flavum, dura, and finally the arachnoid membrane. At this point CSF will flow through the needle if the stylette is withdrawn. The local anesthetic can then be injected and the needle removed. For a paramedian approach the needle is inserted just lateral to the midline and directed slightly medial. In this case the first ligament to be contacted is the ligamentum flavum.

We can adjust the movement of the local anesthetic by making the injected drug lighter (hypobaric), heavier (hyperbaric), or the same density (isobaric) as the CSF, allowing it to float up, sink down, or minimize its spread, respectively.

Spinal anesthesia provides a profound motor and sensory block from a cephalad level (determined by the total dose and the baricity of the drug) caudad to the last sacral nerve roots. It is an excellent choice for all surgeries below mid-abdominal level. For laparoscopic and upper abdominal procedures, diaphragmatic irritation (the diaphragm is innervated by cervical nerves) limits its usefulness. Spinal anesthesia provides more anesthetic area per dose of drug than any other technique (half the body can be anesthetized with 15 mg of bupivacaine or 75 mg of lidocaine). Profound hypotension and bradycardia (even cardiac standstill) can occur quickly, especially if the patient is hypovolemic and the anesthetic level rises above the T4 dermatome. This is caused by blockade of the sympathetic nervous system, which can also cause ptosis and nasal congestion.

The most common complication of spinal anesthesia is postdural puncture headache (5%) which typically comes the day after the subarachnoid puncture. It is positional in nature, getting worse when upright and often completely resolving when recumbent. Leakage of the CSF through the dural puncture site, causing traction on the cranial vessels when the patient becomes upright, is thought to cause the headache. The incidence of headache decreases with age and is less with smaller needles. The type of needle tip also influences headache frequency, with the lowest risk in the pencil point (e.g., Sprotte) needles. Infection (meningitis or abscess), bleeding (epidural hematoma causing cord compression and paralysis), and nerve injury are very rare but devastating complications of spinal anesthesia. Infections at the site of needle placement or prolonged bleeding times are contraindications for central neural blockade.

EPIDURAL AND CAUDAL BLOCKADE

In epidural and caudal anesthesia the needle is not passed through the dura and so may be placed anywhere along the vertebral column without fear of injuring the cord. A specialized needle with a fairly blunt tip is slowly advanced until its tip passes the ligaments of the back and enters the epidural space. Entrance into this potential space is signaled by the ability to inject the contents of a syringe (it is difficult to inject into the ligament and a loss of resistance is felt when leaving it) or the negative pressure caused by the needle tenting the dura and opening the epidural space. Again the needle can be passed midline or paramedian, with the paramedian approach favored in the thoracic region owing to the long and overlapping spinous processes there. Local anesthetic can be injected directly through the needle, but usually a catheter is placed in the epidural space to allow continuous infusions of solution, thus allowing the block to be maintained indefinitely.

The anesthetic solution spreads along the epidural space caudally and cranially with an extent dependent on the volume injected. It usually takes 2 or 3 mL of solution to spread up and down one interspace so 10 mL injected at the L1 interspace will provide a band of anesthesia from T7 to L4 (i.e., from approximately the costal margin to the knees), leaving the sacral dermatomes unaffected. To anesthetize the sacral nerve roots either the catheter can be placed at a low lumbar interspace and large volumes of drug given, or it can be placed via the sacral foramen, in which case the block is often called a caudal block.

The epidural dose of local anesthetic is approximately 10 times greater than the equivalent dose with subarachnoid injection. Because the epidural solution is not mixed with CSF, its concentration once in the epidural space is the same as the injected concentration and is more easily controlled. As each nerve fiber type requires different concentrations to render it nonconductive, the density of the block can be adjusted by using less-concentrated solutions. Lower concentrations will produce loss of autonomic control, temperature sensation, and pain, whereas raising the concentration will eliminate touch, motor strength, and finally proprioception.

Opioids can decrease pain sensation when applied to the spinal cord, usually without affecting its other neural functions, and the combination of a local anesthetic and an opioid has been found to be synergistic in relieving pain. This combination is used in both spinal and epidural anesthesia and is especially useful when treating postoperative or labor pain. By blocking the nerve fibers that transmit painful sensation while sparing motor fibers, the anesthesiologist can allow the patient to be comfortable but still able to push during a delivery or to ambulate.

Postdural puncture headache is rare with epidural anesthesia (0.3%) and is thought to be caused by inadvertent dural puncture. Because the needles used are large, the CSF leak can also be large, producing very intense headaches that require a long time for resolution. If the headache is disabling an epidural puncture can be repeated and the patient's own blood injected into the epidural space. This procedure, called an epidural blood patch, is thought to be effective for two reasons: first, the blood clot formed takes up some space that "replaces" the lost CSF; second, the dural leak is "patched" and the loss of CSF stops. Although this theory of headache and treatment is logical and fits the clinical picture, it has yet to be definitively proven.

As with spinal anesthesia, infection and bleeding are catastrophic complications and must be prevented. Because the epidural needle is often placed in an area where the spinal cord is present in the vertebral canal, advancement of the epidural needle into the canal can cause cord trauma and neurologic injury. There are several techniques for placement that guard against this, and placement above the second lumbar vertebra is performed only by personnel experienced with placement at lower lumbar levels.

PERIPHERAL NERVE BLOCKADE

Of the regional techniques, blockade of the peripheral nerves is possibly the most satisfying and most difficult. The anesthesiologist must be familiar with the anatomy of the area and comparative position of the nerve and surrounding structures and must use an approach that allows the needle to pass to the nerve without damaging vital structures. The underlying principles and techniques are conceptually simple however. In each case the three-dimensional course of the nerve through the area is pictured, and the needle is advanced toward it. The final needle position is determined either by stimulating the nerve with an electric current via the needle tip (causing muscle movement when close to the nerve), by stimulating the nerve by physically touching it with the needle (causing paresthesias), by feeling the needle "pop" into a fascial plane that the nerve is known to be in, or by hitting another structure (e.g., bone or artery) that is known to be in proximity to the nerve. Complications are usually caused either by physically puncturing a structure (e.g., nerve, artery, lung, eye) or by mistakenly placing the local anesthetic solution in an inappropriate place (e.g., intrathecal or intravascular space). Because large volumes of anesthetic are used in some techniques, systemic local anesthetic uptake and toxicity are also possible.

Although spinal and epidural techniques work well for lower extremity surgeries, they are less useful for upper extremity work. This is because the diaphragm and other respiratory muscles are innervated by cervical and thoracic nerves very near the levels of the brachial plexus. It is also unpleasant to have both arms paralyzed and insensate. By blocking the nerves of the brachial plexus, we can cause unilateral upper extremity anesthesia with little respiratory or cardiovascular impairment. These nerves can be blocked in the neck at the interscalene groove (interscalene block), above the first rib (supraclavicular block), below the clavicle (infraclavicular block), in the axilla (axillary block), or in the distal extremity.

Of these the axillary block is the most useful, safest, and most commonly performed. It can provide anesthesia from the axilla distally allowing surgery from the mid-humerus to the fingers. There are no vital structures in the axilla except for the axillary artery, which is quite resistant to injury from puncture. The radial, median, ulnar, and some cutaneous nerves are arranged around the artery, which can be palpated providing a good target. Either the artery can be punctured and the anesthetic delivered behind and in front of it or it can be palpated and the drug placed on either side. In addition a nerve stimulator or a search for paresthesias can be used to provide even more control of the site of injection. The musculocutaneous nerve has often left the sheath that surrounds the nerves and artery at this point. Either it can be anesthetized by injecting enough volume for the drug to spread up the sheath or an injection can be made into the coracobrachialis muscle through which it travels.

The brachial plexus is most compact where it crosses under the clavicle above the first rib and can be completely blocked by a single supraclavicular injection at that point. Unfortunately, it is quite close to the dome of the lung, and care must be taken to keep the first rib between the needle and the lung to avoid pneumothorax.

For procedures at the shoulder, an interscalene injection, which is high in the plexus, is needed. For this block a needle is positioned in the groove between the anterior and middle scalene muscles by either finding a paresthesia or using a nerve stimulator. Care must be taken not to inject into the vertebral artery or into a dural cuff, as the needle will be quite close to the vertebral foramen. This block often misses the C7 and T1 nerve roots of the brachial plexus, which supply much of the ulnar nerve fibers. It is not uncommon to also anesthetize the phrenic nerve (producing unilateral diaphragmatic paralysis) and the stellate ganglion (causing a Horner syndrome).

The nerves of the lower extremity are not as neatly packed as those of the arm. The femoral nerve innervates the anterior muscles of the thigh (quadriceps) and the cutaneous sensation of the anterior thigh and the medial leg to the ankle. The obturator nerve supplies the leg adductors, some sensation to the knee joint, and some sensation to the skin just medial to the knee. The sciatic nerve innervates the posterior thigh muscles, all the muscles below the knee, and the cutaneous sensation of the anterior, lateral, and posterior lower leg. The posterior cutaneous nerve of the thigh runs close to the sciatic nerve in the buttocks and supplies cutaneous sensation to the posterior thigh. Finally, the lateral femoral cutaneous nerve supplies cutaneous sensation to the lateral thigh. Although full anesthesia requires blockade of all of these nerves, in practice we can usually be selective about where blockade is needed.

The femoral nerve is easily found just lateral to the femoral artery distal to the inguinal ligament and can be located with paresthesias or a nerve stimulator. Typically the obturator nerve is blocked as part of a "three-in-one" block of the femoral nerve. Here a large volume of anesthetic solution is injected into the femoral nerve sheath. If pressure is put on the sheath distal to the injection site, the solution will flow proximally and bathe the obturator and lateral femoral cutaneous nerve as well. An isolated obturator nerve block can be performed, but it is rarely needed without a femoral block and so is rarely done. The lateral femoral cutaneous nerve can be blocked just above the inguinal ligament and is useful for pain relief after skin grafting. Patients with quadriceps weakness from a femoral block have difficulty using crutches as they cannot keep their leg straight or keep it from swinging. Because of this, prolonged femoral nerve blocks can delay discharge of ambulatory patients.

Sciatic nerve block can be accomplished at many sites, including the lower medial quadrant of the buttocks (Labat's approach), between the ischial tuberosity and the greater trochanter (in the lithotomy position), and either anteriorly or laterally as the nerve courses through the thigh behind the femur. The popliteal block is just a sciatic block at a point approximately 5 cm above the popliteal crease as the nerve is dividing into the tibial and common peroneal nerves. These blocks are very safe as they cause little cardiovascular change and have few vital structures near the nerve to injure. They nicely anesthetize the tissue of the entire lower extremity except for the skin, which can be infiltrated at the surgical site. A patient with a full sciatic nerve block can easily ambulate with crutches because they retain strength in the quadriceps and so can control their knee movement.

In addition one can block the nerves of the face, neck, hands, and ankles. The nerves of the trunk can also be blocked either just as they leave the spinal canal or, in the case of the chest, as intercostal nerves. Thus there are as many nerve blocks as there are nerves in the body.

BIER BLOCK

IV regional blockade was first described by August Bier in 1908 and is still a widely used technique today. It is partly a local anesthetic technique and partly a regional one inasmuch as it uses the veins to spread local anesthetic over the whole extremity. After a small IV catheter is placed distally, an elastic bandage (Esmarch) or gravity is used to empty the extremity of blood, and a proximal tourniquet is inflated to one to two times the systolic blood pressure. A local anesthetic solution is then injected into the IV catheter, and anesthesia is rapidly produced distal to the tourniquet. This block is easy, reliable, and quick and is useful for short procedures of the hand and lower leg. Because the tissue directly under the tourniquet is not anesthetized, tourniquet pain is noted after 30 to 60 minutes.

SUMMARY

This chapter has described the basics of regional anesthesia and the use of local anesthetics. It is an exciting field of anesthesia, fun to do, and safe, and can be used to provide surgical anesthesia and pain relief to many patients, including those in the operative suite, the recovery area, the emergency room, labor and delivery, and the pain clinic.

SUGGESTED READINGS

Cousins MJ, Bridenbaugh PO. Neural Blockade in Clinical Anesthesia and Management of Pain, 3rd Ed. Baltimore: Lippincott Williams & Wilkins, 1997.

Miller RD. Anesthesia, 4th Ed. New York: Churchill Livingstone, 1994, pp 1535–1594.

Scott DB. Techniques of Regional Anaesthesia. 2nd Ed. Norwalk, Conn.: Appleton & Lange/Mediglobe, 1995.

CHAPTER 6

Perioperative Monitoring

Mark E. Comunale, MD

Monitoring is an essential part of an anesthesiologist's duties. Because anesthesia, surgery, and concomitant disease can cause rapid changes in a patient's physiologic condition, it is necessary for the anesthesiologist to continuously assess the patient immediately before, during, and immediately after anesthesia. Monitoring serves to detect such changes, which, if left uncorrected, could potentially lead to adverse consequences.

Anesthesia monitoring involves both qualitative and quantitative assessment of the patient. Qualitative assessment is performed using the senses of sight, sound, and touch. Quantitative assessment uses instruments designed to measure physiologic functions. Both types of monitoring allow rapid assessment of information and response to changes in the patient's physiologic state.

Minimal monitoring standards (known as "Harvard Minimal Monitoring Standards") were first established at Beth Israel Hospital, Boston in 1985.[1] The American Society of Anesthesiologists subsequently established similar standards for basic anesthetic monitoring in 1986. These minimal monitoring standards (Table 6-1) are applied to all patients undergoing anesthesia.

CIRCULATORY SYSTEM

Pulse

A superficial pulse can be palpated in a number of areas. Common sites used during anesthesia are radial, superficial temporal, carotid, and facial arteries. This latter site is convenient when administering mask anesthesia, as one finger of the hand holding the mask can be used to palpate the pulse of the facial artery where it crosses the mandible. Palpation of the pulse allows both quantitative (heart rate) and qualitative (strength of pulsation as an estimate of blood pressure) evaluation of the circulatory status.

A pulse plethysmograph is an alternative method of obtaining the pulse. This instrument senses tissue blood volume by the attenuation of light emitted from and detected by a probe that is placed over an extremity (finger, toe, earlobe, or nose). Blood entering and leaving the extremity causes pulsatile increases and decreases in the volume of the extremity. If light is passed through the extremity, absorption of light will occur causing variable intensity with each pulse wave. The variable intensity of light is detected by the instrument and converted to an electrical signal whose

51

Table 6-1. Minimal Monitoring Standards for Anesthesia

1. Qualified anesthesia personnel will be present throughout the conduct of all general, regional, and monitored anesthesia care.

2. During all anesthetics, the patient's oxygenation, ventilation, circulation, and temperature shall be continually evaluated.

3. Oxygenation

   A. During the administration of anesthesia using an anesthesia machine, the concentration of oxygen in the patient breathing system shall be measured using an oxygen analyzer with a low oxygen concentration limit alarm in use.

   B. During all anesthetics, a quantitative method of assessing oxygenation such as pulse oximetry shall be used. Adequate illumination and exposure of the patient are necessary to assess color.

4. Ventilation

   A. Adequacy of ventilation shall be continually evaluated in every patient receiving general anesthesia. In addition to clinical science such as chest excursion, observation of the reservoir breathing bag, and auscultation of breath sounds, quantitative monitoring of the carbon dioxide content and volume of expired gas is strongly encouraged.

   B. When an endotracheal tube is inserted, its presence in the trachea must be verified by clinical assessment and by identification of carbon dioxide in the expired gas. Continual end-tidal carbon dioxide analysis shall be performed using quantitative methods such as capnography, capnometry, or mass spectroscopy from the time of endotracheal tube placement until extubation or initiating transfer to a postoperative care location.

   C. During mechanical ventilation, a device that is capable of detecting disconnection of the components of breathing system shall be in continuous use. This device will have an audible signal when its alarm threshold is exceeded.

   D. During regional anesthesia and monitored anesthesia care, adequacy of ventilation shall be evaluated at minimum by continual observation of qualitative clinical science.

5. Circulation

   A. All patients receiving anesthesia shall have the electrocardiogram continuously displayed from the beginning of anesthesia until preparing to leave the anesthetizing location.

   B. All patients receiving anesthesia shall have arterial blood pressure and heart rate determined, evaluated, and recorded at least every 5 minutes.

   C. All patients receiving general anesthesia shall have, in addition to the above, circulatory function continually evaluated by at least one of the following: palpation of a pulse, auscultation of heart sounds, monitoring of a trace of intra-arterial pressure, ultrasound, peripheral pulse monitoring, or pulse plethysmography or oximetry.

6. Body Temperature

   A. A means to continuously measure the patient's temperature shall be readily available for all patients. Body temperature shall be measured when changes in body temperature are intended, anticipated, or suspected.

Adapted from *Standards for Basic Anesthetic Monitoring.* Approved by the American Society of Anesthesiologists House of Delegates on October 21, 1986, and last amended on October 21, 1998.

Table 6-1 is reprinted with permission of the American Society of Anesthesiologists, 520 N. Northwest Highway, Park Ridge, Illinois 60068-2573.

amplitude is proportional to blood volume in the extremity (blood flow) and whose frequency is proportional to heart rate. In modern anesthesia, a pulse oximeter is a pulse plethysmograph combined with an infrared light source and detector. This instrument is capable of quantitatively measuring pulse and oxygen saturation of hemoglobin in the extremity.[2,3]

Pulse may also be qualitatively and quantitatively measured by the use of an arterial catheter (see "Invasive Monitoring").

Blood Pressure

The arterial pressure pulse is very complex, being composed of both a pressure wave (propagated at 5 to 10 m/sec) and a flow element (conducted as a much slower average velocity of 0.3 to 0.5 m/sec). The pressure pulse is generated by the mechanical contractions of the heart and sustained by the viscoelastic properties of the arteries. As such, the pressure pulse is markedly changed as it travels distally through the body, undergoing amplification and contour transformation.[4] Also, the flow velocity drops dramatically as the cross-section of the vascular system increases from the aorta to the capillaries.[5,6] This alteration of pressure pulse from the arch of the aorta to the distal arterioles explains some of the variability in blood pressure obtained by different methods and different arterial locations.

Indirect Pressure Measurements

The blood pressure cuff is wrapped around an extremity and inflated with air, collapsing the underlying artery. The pressure within the cuff is assumed to equal that of the arterial vessel wall. As the cuff is slowly deflated for a series of pulses, cuff pressure is continually noted. Simultaneously, a signal of interest is observed (arterial line pulsation, Korotkoff sounds, oscillation in cuff pressure; Fig. 6-1). Cuff size is important in obtaining accurate indirect blood pressure measurements. The best cuff width is approximately 40% of the circumference of the arm.[7] This will allow a uniform pressure to develop around the limb. Narrower cuffs do not produce a uniform pressure increase throughout the underlying extremity segment and cause inaccurate determination of blood pressure. A cuff less than 40% of arm circumference will give readings higher than actual arterial wall pressure.[8] It is always better to ere on the side of using a cuff that is too large, as the error introduced by too large a cuff is minimal. Wrapping the blood pressure cuff loosely or eccentrically will allow part of the inflated cuff to lift off the skin, and a similar artifact is produced.

Electrocardiogram

It is important to recognize that the electrocardiogram (ECG) provides information about electrical activity and not mechanical activity of the heart. The ECG is useful in obtaining information regarding cardiac rhythm and rate. The ECG must be continuously displayed and monitored during the conduct of an anesthetic. Modern anesthesia monitors, which display the ECG, also indicate each QRS complex with an audible tone. Thus, the anesthesiologist

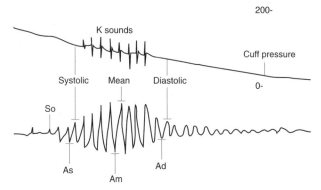

FIGURE 6-1. Oscillometric measurement of blood pressure as compared with Korotkoff sounds (K sounds). So, the initial point of cuff oscillation; As, auscultatory systolic pressure; Am, auscultatory mean blood pressure; Ad, point at which diastolic blood pressure would be read by auscultation. (Redrawn with permission from Reitan JA, Barash PG, Noninvasive monitoring. In Saidman LJ, Smith NT, eds: Monitoring in Anesthesia. Stoneham, Butterworth, 1984. p124.

is able to perform other tasks without having to continuously observe the ECG. The combination of an audible QRS indicator and an audible pulse plethysmograph tone allows continuous monitoring of electrical and mechanical activity of the heart when not looking at the display screen.

In addition to arrhythmia detection, another important function of the ECG is as a monitor of myocardial ischemia. Although it is not practical nor possible to monitor a continuous 12-lead ECG during anesthesia, London and colleagues determined that the 3-lead combination of leads 2, V_5, and V_4 had a 96% sensitivity in detecting ischemia when compared with the 12-lead ECG.[9] Although criteria for diagnosing myocardial ischemia vary, myocardial ischemia is generally accepted as ST-segment depression of at least 1 mm (0. mV from baseline) measured at the J point + 60 msec in any lead lasting at least 1 minute.[10,11] Many monitors have filters that prevent electrocautery interference on the ECG. To detect myocardial ischemia, an ECG monitor must have a bandwidth as low as 0.05 Hz. Many electrocautery filters attenuate the bandwidth to 0.5 Hz, thus preventing diagnosis of myocardial ischemia.[12]

OXYGENATION AND VENTILATION

Pulse Oximetry

A pulse oximeter is an instrument that combines a pulse plethysmograph with technology capable of measuring oxygen saturation of hemoglobin. The pulse oximeter works by projecting light of near infrared wavelength

(660 nm) and infrared wavelength (910 or 940 nm) through tissue of an extremity such as a finger or an earlobe. The light transmitted is decreased by absorption of tissues other than blood. With each pulse, the amount of light is also decreased by the amount of deoxyhemoglobin and oxyhemoglobin in the arterial blood that enters the extremity. The remaining light transmitted through the extremity is detected by a photodiode. Because the specific absorptions of tissue and blood are known, only the concentrations of deoxyhemoglobin and oxyhemoglobin remain as variables. The percent saturation of hemoglobin (SpO_2) is then displayed as a numerical value on the monitor.

The pulse oximeter continually provides important information to the anesthesiologist. Not only does the pulse plethysmograph provide confirmation of the mechanical activity of the heart, but continuous measurement of oxygen saturation allows prompt evaluation and intervention during times when oxygenation is compromised and SpO_2 falls. Like the audible QRS tone on the ECG monitor, pulse oximeters are equipped with an audible tone generated by the pulse plethysmograph. Unlike the audible tone for the QRS complex on the ECG, the pulse oximeter tone changes with each 1% change in oxygen saturation. This audible signal with changing tone allows the anesthesiologist to perform other tasks while continuously monitoring hemoglobin saturation when not looking directly at the monitors. Experienced anesthesiologists are capable of detecting the change in tone caused by a 1% decrease in arterial hemoglobin saturation. A number of factors interfere with the accuracy of the pulse oximeter including fingernail polish, ambient light, abnormal hemoglobins, operation of electrosurgical units, movement, and various dyes.[2]

End-Tidal Capnography

During anesthesia, exhaled CO_2 from the patient is measured and numerically and graphically displayed on the patient monitors. CO_2 can be measured using infrared spectrometry, Raman spectrometry, mass spectrometry, and photoacoustic spectrometry.[13] In all cases, CO_2 is sampled from the breathing circuit as close as possible to the endotracheal tube. End-tidal capnography allows the anesthesiologist to monitor a number of important variables during anesthesia. In patients without significant lung disease, the end-tidal CO_2 value displayed on the capnograph correlates closely with values for carbon dioxide obtained by arterial blood gas sampling. End-tidal capnography therefore provides a noninvasive measure of adequacy of ventilation during general anesthesia. The capnograph displays a plot of expired CO_2 concentration versus time or exhaled volume.

Changes in exhaled CO_2 tension or waveform can be used to detect acute changes in cardiac output, airway obstruction, pulmonary embolus, esophageal intubation, and onset of malignant hyperthermia.[14] Figure 6-2 shows examples of changes expected in exhaled CO_2 tension and waveform associated with various conditions.

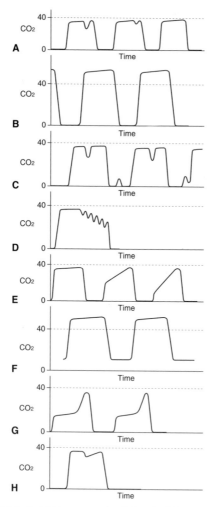

FIGURE 6-2. End-tidal capnography during the following conditions: curare notch or residual neuromuscular blockade effect (the third example shows a complete reversal; (A) hypoventilation or increased CO_2 production (B); spontaneous respiration during mechanical ventilation (C); cardiac oscillation (D); bronchospasm (E); rebreathing (F); sample tube leak (G); and substantial difference in compliance between lungs (H).

Ventilatory Flow and Volume

Expired gas volume is measured directly using a variety of flowmeters called spirometers. Spirometers are an adaptation of the instrument originally introduced by Wright.[15] The spirometer or volume meter is attached to the expiratory limb of the anesthesia breathing circuit and measures the volume of gas expired in spontaneously breathing patients and in patients who are mechanically ventilated. Expired gas volume is displayed as either tidal volume of each breath or, when multiplied by respiratory rate, as minute ventilation. In addition to qualitative measures of ventilation such as observing respiratory movements of the chest wall, condensation in the endotracheal tube, or movement of the breathing bag or ventilator bellows, the volume meter on the anesthesia machine provides a quantitative estimate of ventilation. Many volume meters are equipped with an audible alarm, which is triggered when low flow or no flow occurs for greater than 1 minute. Thus, volume meters can be helpful in detecting circuit disconnects and leaks.

During mask anesthesia in a spontaneously breathing patient, a sudden increase in tidal volume as can be observed on the volume meter often occurs before changes in heart rate or blood pressure in response to surgical stimuli.

Airway Pressure

Airway pressure is measured by a pressure gauge on the inspiratory limb of the breathing circuit. Peak inspiratory pressure is a useful monitoring variable during anesthesia and depends on the resistance to flow in the breathing system and the compliance of chest wall, lungs, and breathing circuit. In normal healthy patients, peak inspiratory pressures generally range from 5 to 30 cm H_2O. Increases and decreases in peak inspiratory pressures provide information on the status of the breathing circuit, and compliance of lungs and chest wall. For example, increases in peak inspiratory pressures can be caused by bronchospasm, breathing circuit obstruction, or increased intra-abdominal pressure as occurs during laparoscopic surgery. Decreases in peak inspiratory pressures can be caused by leaks in the breathing system, use of extremely compliant breathing circuits, or inadequate inspiratory flow rate on the ventilator.

TEMPERATURE MONITORING

Temperature measurement capability should be available in all anesthetizing locations. Most anesthesiologists use temperature probes designed to fit in the nasopharynx or posterior oropharynx. Temperature monitoring is critical for the prevention of hypothermia during anesthesia and surgery as well as for the detection of malignant hyperthermia in response to anesthesia and stress.

Hypothermia can have serious consequences for patients undergoing anesthesia and surgery. Body heat loss can occur as a result of exposure to cool operating rooms (21°C), evaporative heat loss from skin surfaces, and conduction of heat to cooler objects in contact with the body.[16] Hypothermia depresses cerebral function, causing delayed awakening from anesthesia or prolonged neuromuscular blockade.[17] Postoperative shivering in the hypothermic patient can increase oxygen consumption by 100%, increasing both cardiac output and minute ventilation.[18] These responses may have serious consequences in patients who are hypovolemic or who have coronary artery disease. Hypothermia can interfere with hemostasis because many proteins necessary for adequate coagulation lose function in a hypothermic environment.

Hypothermia is most easily prevented by active warming of the patient through the use of warming blankets and intravenous fluid warmers.

MONITORING FLUID HOMEOSTASIS

Monitoring fluid homeostasis during anesthesia takes into account a number of factors such as length of time the patient has been without food and water before anesthesia, invasiveness of the surgical procedure, site of surgical procedure, potential for blood loss during the procedure, and urine output. If a urinary catheter is used, the measurement of urine output also provides an indication of fluid status. In general, a urine output of at least 0.5 mL/kg per hour is acceptable during anesthesia and surgery and indicates adequate fluid homeostasis. Small amounts of dark, concentrated urine suggest hypovolemia. The appearance of red-tinged urine can be caused by traumatic catheter insertion or, more importantly, hemoglobinemia from blood transfusion reaction. Management of perioperative fluid and blood replacement is beyond the scope of this chapter. Please refer to Chapter 9 for an in-depth discussion of perioperative fluid management.

INVASIVE MONITORING

Invasive monitoring is indicated when the patient's physiologic condition or procedures affecting the patient's physiologic condition have the potential to change rapidly or when the patient's underlying disease state is such that rapid continuous assessment of vital signs and management is necessary.

Arterial Catheters: Direct Blood Pressure Measurement

Blood pressure can be measured directly from a fluid-filled catheter through insertion into an artery. In anesthesia, common sites for direct arterial pressure measurement are the radial and femoral arteries. The catheter is connected to fluid-filled tubing and a pressure transducer. Pressure transducers are electromechanical devices that change pressure energy into an electrical potential. The transducer consists of a transducer membrane and electronic components. The intravascular pressure wave generates a slight to and fro motion in the connecting tubing that deforms the transducer membrane and produces electrical voltage.

Before interpreting the pressures derived from the pressure pulse, the transducer must be zeroed. Intravascular pressures are not specified as absolute pressures but are referenced or measured as a difference from the atmospheric pressure surrounding the body. Pressures within both the arterial and venous system reflect not just the pressure pulse of cardiac ejection but also the hydrostatic pressure (gravitational energy) of the vertical offset of the transducer above or below the heart. By convention, intravascular pressures are referenced to atmosphere at the atrial level. As long as the relative vertical distance between the heart and the transducer remains unchanged, the zeroing of the transducer remains valid.

The physiologic monitor amplifies, filters, and processes the transducer's signal and displays the pressure waveform. Current physiologic monitors also display in digital form the systolic, mean, and diastolic pressures.

Central Venous Pressure

Central venous access is often necessary during volume resuscitation, and is useful for air embolus removal and administration of vasoactive and inotropic drugs. In general, the central venous pressure (CVP) will reflect left atrial pressure and can serve as a surrogate for pulmonary capillary wedge pressure (PCWP) in patients with normal lungs.

For central access and measurement of CVP, a catheter can be inserted through the external jugular, internal jugular, or subclavian vein. The catheter is advanced until its tip lies in the distal superior vena cava just above the right atrium. To obtain information about the patient's volume status, the anesthesiologist connects the central venous line to a pressure transducer and displays a CVP tracing on a patient care monitor. In normal sinus rhythm, the characteristic CVP tracing with *a, c,* and *v* waves and *x* and *y* descents can be observed (Fig. 6-3). The mean CVP can then be used as a guide in evaluating patient volume status and management of fluid therapy.

Pulmonary Artery Catheters

Pulmonary artery (PA) catheters are used to monitor volume status and cardiac output and, in conjunction with other monitors, for the detection of myocardial ischemia. Current PA catheters may have additional functions

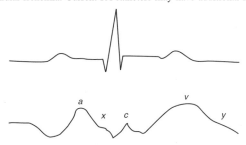

FIGURE 6-3. Central venous pressure tracing (bottom) relative to electrocardiographic tracing (top). *a* wave, atrial systole; *c* wave, bulging of tricuspid valve back toward atrium during ventricular systole; *v* wave, passive right atrial filling. Note that mechanical activity occurs slightly after electrocardiogram electrical activity.

such as the measurement of mixed venous oxygen saturation or pacing capability. However, all PA catheters currently used have the following common characteristics: a distal lumen for the measurement of PA pressure, a proximal lumen for the measurement of CVP, an inflatable balloon at the distal end of the catheter for flow-directed placement and to obtain PCWP, and a thermistor, also located at the distal end of the catheter, which is used for measuring core temperature and cardiac output.

PA catheters can be inserted through the internal or external jugular vein, subclavian vein, or femoral vein. Most commonly, the internal jugular venous route is used.

The PA catheter is connected to pressure transducers to measure central venous and PA pressures. After placement of an introducer sheath into the internal jugular vein, the PA catheter is introduced through the sheath. The balloon at the end of the catheter is inflated to allow flow-directed advancement through the right atrium, across the tricuspid valve, through the right ventricle, across the pulmonary valve, and into the PA to obtain the PCWP. As the catheter is advanced from right atrium to PA, characteristic waveforms are observed (Fig. 6-4). A number of hemodynamic measurements useful for patient management may be obtained using the PA catheter. Cardiac output may be measured via the thermodilution method, and is obtained by injecting a known volume of fluid at a known temperature (4°C

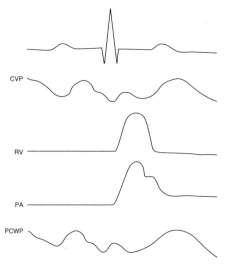

FIGURE 6-4. Characteristic pressure waveforms during pulmonary artery (PA) line placement relative to electrocardiographic tracing (top). Advancement of catheter tip through right atrium (CVP), into right ventricle (RV), into PA, and into pulmonary capillary wedge position (PCWP).

or 21°C) into the right atrium through the CVP port of the PA catheter. The change in temperature associated with the bolus of fluid is detected in the PA by the thermistor at the distal end of the PA catheter. A computer then integrates the area under the curve of temperature versus time and calculates the cardiac output. PA catheters are useful in the management of patients who are critically ill or who have the potential to become critically ill as a result of their surgery. Some examples of the way a PA catheter may be used to manage a patient are shown in Table 6-2.

Table 6-2. Hemodynamics in Diagnosis and Management

MAP	CVP	PA	PCWP	CO	SVR	Diagnosis	Treatment
low	high	high	high	low	high	congestive heart failure	combined inotropic agent, vasodilator (e.g., dobutamine)
low	low	low	low	low	high	hypovolemia	volume replacement
low	low/nl	low/nl	low/nl	high	low	vasodilation	vasoconstrictor
high	nl	nl	nl	nl/low	high	hypertensive	vasodilator

MAP, mean arterial pressure; CVP, central venous pressure; PA, pulmonary artery pressure; PCWP, pulmonary capillary wedge pressure; CO, cardiac output; SVR, systemic vascular resistance = (MAP − CVP/CO) × 80 dyne · sec · cm-5; nl, normal.

SUMMARY

Monitoring during and immediately after anesthesia is an essential part of an anesthesiologist's duties. Continuous monitoring of respiratory, cardiac, and other physiologic functions allows the anesthesiologist to rapidly assess and respond to changes in the patient's condition caused by anesthesia or surgery.

Monitoring standards have been developed and used during all anesthetics and include monitoring oxygenation, ventilation, circulatory status, and body temperature.

REFERENCES

1. Eichhorn JH, Cooper JB, Cullen DJ, et al. Standards for patient monitoring during anesthesia at Harvard Medical School. JAMA 1986;256:1017-1021.
2. Kelleher JR. Pulse oximetry. J Clin Monit 1989;5:37-62.
3. Tremper KK, Barker SJ. Pulse oximetry. Anesthesiology 1989;70:98-108.
4. Bruner JM, Krenis LG, Kunsman JM, et al. Comparison of direct and indirect methods of measuring arterial blood pressure: part II. Med Instrum 1981;15:97-101.
5. Hamilton WF, Woodbury RA, Harper HT. Optical tracing of human blood pressure, comparing critical and oscillographic criteria with the true blood pressure. Am J Physiol 1936;113:59.
6. Prys-Roberts C. Measurement of intravascular pressure. In: Saidman LJ, Smith 1978;68-72. NT, eds. Monitoring in Anesthesia. New York: Churchill Livingstone, 1978.
7. Geddes LA. The Direct and Indirect Measurement of Blood Pressure. Chicago: Year Book Medical Publishers, 1970.
8. Simpson JA, Jamieson G, Dickhaus DW, Grover RF. Effect of size of cuff bladder on accuracy of measurement of indirect blood pressure. Am Heart J 1965;70:208-215.
9. London MJ, Hollenber M, Wong MG, et al. Intraoperative myocardial ischemia: localization by continuous 12-lead electrocardiography. Anesthesiology 1988;69:232-241.
10. Knight AA, Hollenberg M, London MJ, et al. Perioperative myocardial ischemia: importance of the preoperative ischemic pattern. Anesthesiology 1988;68:681-688.
11. Cohen M, Scharpf SS, Rentrop KP. Prospective analysis of electrocardiographic variables as markers for extent and location of acute wall motion abnormalities observed during coronary angioplasty in human subjects. J Am Coll Cardiol 1987;10:17-24.
12. Subcommittee on Exercise Testing. Guidelines for exercise testing. J Am Coll Cardiol 1986;8:725-738.
13. Bhavi-Shankar K, Mosley H, Kumar AY, Delph Y. Capnometry and anaesthesia. Can J Anaesth 1992;39:617-632.
14. Sackner MA, Krieger BP. Noninvasive respiratory monitoring. In: Scharf SM, Cassidy SS, eds. Heart Lung Interactions in Health and Disease. New York: Marcel Dekker, 1989;663-792
15. Wright BM. A respiratory anemometer. J Physiol (Lond) 1955;127:25P.
16. Ryan JF. Unintentional hypothermia. In: Orkin FK, Cooperman LH, eds. Complications in Anesthesiology. Philadelphia: JB Lippincott, 1983; 284-291.

17. Cork RC. Temperature monitoring. In: Blite CD, Hines RL, eds. Monitoring in Anesthesia and Critical Care, 3rd ed. New York: Churchill Livingstone, 1995;441-457.
18. Vaughan MS, Vaughan RW, Cork RC. Postoperative hypothermia in adults: relationship of age, anesthesia and shivering to rewarming. Anesth Analg 1981;60:746-751.

CHAPTER 7

Intravenous Sedation

David C. Lai, MD

INTRODUCTION

Intravenous sedation is an anesthetic technique that is commonly used (1) as a prelude to regional or general anesthesia, (2) in conjunction with regional anesthesia, or (3) as an anesthetic adjunct to provide for patient comfort when local anesthesia is administered by the surgeon. All anesthesiologists are trained to provide intravenous sedation, but not all intravenous sedation is provided by trained anesthesiologists. This is an important distinction, as intravenous sedation can potentially be extremely challenging, requiring the skills and knowledge of an experienced anesthesiologist. Because non-anesthesiologists often give intravenous sedation outside of the operating room, it is an important skill for all physicians to learn.

DEFINITION

Intravenous sedation is any medication administered intravenously that may change one's mental state. On the other hand, general anesthesia is an induced mental state in which the patient is unconscious. Patients may refer to this as "being knocked out" or "totally asleep." Although general anesthesia usually necessitates an airway adjunct, such as an endotracheal tube or a laryngeal mask airway (LMA), the patient may require only a face mask (mask general anesthesia) with or without nasal or oral airways.

When intravenous sedation is used, a continuum exists between the conscious and unconscious states. The moment a sedated patient becomes unconscious, the anesthetic technique becomes intravenous general anesthesia, carrying with it all the attendant risks and considerations of a general anesthetic. Although both cardiovascular and respiratory complications may occur, airway compromise is by far the most common problem. The respiratory efforts of an unconscious patient may vary from adequate spontaneous breathing to various degrees of airway obstruction. If the patient is at risk for aspiration (e.g., full stomach, hiatal hernia, gastroesophageal reflux disease), then they should not be having the equivalent of general anesthesia without a protected airway. If the patient is no longer breathing (apneic), or if airway obstruction does not allow effective oxygenation and ventilation, hypoxic brain damage and cardiovascular disturbance may occur unless effective oxygenation and ventilation are restored. This underscores the importance of the individual administering intravenous sedation being capable of establishing a patent airway and providing positive-pressure ventilation if necessary.

MONITORED ANESTHESIA CARE

Intravenous sedation provided by anesthesiologists is often referred to as monitored anesthesia care, or MAC (not to be confused with minimum alveolar concentration MAC). We often choose this technique for patients who do not require a general or regional anesthetic technique, but who need more than just local anesthesia for comfort.

Conceptually, MAC is attractive because it usually does not involve airway manipulations other than chin lift, jaw thrust, or a nasal or oral airway, and it usually produces fewer physiologic perturbations. It is therefore considered a safe and attractive option for patients who are at increased risk for general or regional anesthesia, or are afraid of "needles in the back" or "going to sleep." Although such an assumption is often true, we will see later that it is not always the case.

The term MAC was intended to replace the inaccurate and now defunct term of "local/standby." Local/standby arose during an era when anesthesiologists were asked to be available to stand by to provide monitoring and sedation for high-risk patients too sick to undergo general anesthesia. A classic example was a patient with multiple-organ failure undergoing tracheostomy. To more clearly delineate the anesthesiologist's role in the management of such patients, the American Society of Anesthesiologists defined MAC in 1986 as: "... instances in which an anesthesiologist has been called upon to provide specific anesthesia services to a particular patient undergoing a planned procedure, in connection with which a patient receives local anesthesia, or in some cases, no anesthesia at all. In such a case, the anesthesiologist is providing specific services to the patient and is in control of the patient's non-surgical or non-obstetric medical care, including the responsibility of monitoring the patient's vital signs, and is available to administer anesthetics or provide other medical care as appropriate." The anesthesiologist, acting as the patient's perioperative physician, performs a preoperative assessment and uses intraoperative monitoring, but does not necessarily administer any medications.

Just as local/standby is a misnomer, local/MAC can also be misleading. "Monitored" anesthesia care implies that there is "unmonitored" anesthesia care. All anesthetic care is monitored—whether it is MAC, regional, or general anesthesia. In addition, all anesthetic care—including MAC—necessitates an anesthesiologist's preoperative anesthetic assessment and his or her presence during the procedure.

CONSCIOUS SEDATION

The term "conscious sedation" has often been used to describe sedation and analgesia given by non-anesthesiologists to patients undergoing diagnostic or therapeutic procedures. The goal is to relieve a patient's anxiety or pain, and make uncomfortable situations more tolerable without compromising safety.

The American Dental Association first introduced the term conscious sedation to describe sedation or analgesia administered for dental procedures. They defined conscious sedation as a "depressed level of consciousness that allows the patient the ability to independently and continuously maintain an airway and respond appropriately to physical stimulation and verbal command," and deep sedation (hypnosis) as a "controlled state of depressed consciousness accompanied by partial or complete loss of protective reflexes, including the ability to independently maintain an airway and respond purposefully to physical stimulation or verbal command." Deep sedation as defined above is really a description of general anesthesia. Loss of protective reflexes, loss of airway, and lack of purposeful response to stimulation are all hallmarks of the unconscious state, i.e., general anesthesia.

Vigilance must constantly be maintained, as too much conscious sedation may lead to unconscious sedation — the dental deep sedation. Even a little unconscious sedation may potentially lead to big problems — cardiac or respiratory depression that may lead to hypoxic brain damage, cardiac arrest, or death. Although one strives to maintain conscious sedation, this may not always be possible given the rapidity with which patients may move between being conscious and unconscious.

The US Food and Drug Administration further defined (or confused) different levels of sedation as (1) pre-procedural sedation, (2) conscious sedation, (3) deep sedation, and (4) general anesthesia. As we have seen above, these distinctions are often hard to make.

Sedation or analgesia is therefore the appropriate term to describe care provided by both anesthesiologists and non-anesthesiologists. Anesthesiologists, however, can safely provide care that goes beyond conscious sedation, whereas non-anesthesiologists usually cannot. Non-anesthesiologists should restrict themselves to lighter levels of sedation or analgesia, and defer to the anesthesiologist when the procedures or patients require heavier degrees of sedation or analgesia. Table 7-1 compares conscious sedation with deep sedation, with the understanding that deep sedation really refers to general anesthesia with an unprotected airway. (This type of anesthetic state is often euphemistically termed GANA, short for general anesthesia—no airway!)

PHARMACOLOGY

The drugs most commonly administered during intravenous sedation include benzodiazepines (midazolam), opioids (fentanyl, remifentanil), and sedative hypnotics (propofol, methohexital, ketamine) (see Chapter 4). It is important to realize that all of these agents have the ability to cause cardiac and respiratory depression, but are relatively safe when used alone and in titrated amounts. Increased dosage and frequency of these drugs, especially when used concomitantly, increase the chance for cardiac and respiratory depression. Other factors to consider when using these drugs include opioid-induced pruritus (commonly the nose), disinhibition (patients may become very talkative), and paradoxical reactions (patients may become unruly and agitated).

Table 7-1. A Comparison of the Important Features of an Ideal Conscious Sedation Technique and a Deep Sedation Technique

Conscious Sedation	Deep Sedation
Verbal communication possible	Verbal communication impossible
Patient can cooperate	No patient cooperation
Patient reassurance possible	Unrecognized respiratory insufficiency more likely
May monitor cardiorespiratory and neurologic status	No monitor of neurologic status
Airway reflexes intact	Airway reflexes attenuated
Aspiration unlikely	Aspiration possible
Airway dilator muscles functional	Airway dilator muscles dysfunctional
Obstruction unlikely	Obstruction likely
Normal work of breathing	Increased work of breathing
Severe hypoventilation less likely	Hypoventilation likely
Respiratory control relatively intact	Respiratory control attenuated
Hypoxia or hypercarbia less likely	Hypoxia or hypercarbia likely
Patient able to maintain own airway	Patient unable to maintain own airway
Need for unplanned intubation or other airway intervention unlikely	Unplanned intubation or airway intervention likely
Respiratory complications unlikely	Respiratory complications likely
	Hypoventilation
	Aspiration
	Obstruction
	Postobstructive pulmonary edema
	Airway instrumentation
	Failed intubation
	Cannot ventilate or oxygenate scenario
	Hypoxic neurologic damage
	Delayed recovery with possible morbidity

Adapted with permission from Hillier SC. Monitored anesthesia care. In: Barash PG, Cullen, BF, Stoelting RK, eds. Clinical Anesthesia. 3rd Ed. Philadelphia: Lippincott-Raven, 1996.

One must balance the tasks of titrating drugs and allowing time for their mental status effects to equilibrate while assessing and reassessing quickly changing surgical stimuli. This is often a challenging task and a potential source of complications. The hallmark of a good anesthesiologist is one who can make this look effortless, belying the training and experience that makes it possible. The art of anesthesia is in making the difficult appear easy.

SURGICAL PROCEDURES COMMONLY PERFORMED UNDER INTRAVENOUS SEDATION

Procedures performed with intravenous sedation fall into three categories: (1) procedures using sedation with or without topical anesthesia, such as extracorporeal shock wave lithotripsy, computerized tomography, magnetic resonance imaging, ocular surgery, upper or lower gastrointestinal endoscopic examinations, cardiac catheterizations, bronchoscopies, various minor procedures; (2) procedures using sedation and local anesthetic infiltration or blocks, such as vascular access, ocular surgery, excisions, herniorrhaphy, dilation and curettage, podiatry; and (3) procedures using sedation and regional anesthesia, such as spinal, epidural, or brachial plexus blocks.

TECHNIQUES

Intravenous sedation/analgesia may be given either as a bolus, an infusion, or a combination of both. We can control the rate of administration using an infusion pump, or by the experienced hand of the anesthesiologist. If the surgeon is injecting local anesthesia, we usually give the patient sedation or analgesia before the injection, with the peak effect hopefully coinciding with the onset and duration of the noxious stimuli. Timing and dose are critical for both patient comfort and safety. If the peak effect is too late or not adequate, the patient will experience discomfort. If the peak effect comes too late or is overly generous for a given stimulus the patient is at risk for cardiac or respiratory compromise. Such untoward effects must be recognized promptly, and appropriate measures taken.

Further sedation or analgesia must be tempered against constantly changing requirements. It is often unclear whether a patient needs more sedation, or more local anesthetic infiltration. One approach to this is to carefully sedate the patient to the point where they are audibly snoring (often easier said than done). This serves two purposes: (1) it is irrefutable proof to everyone in the operating room that the patient is indeed asleep, sedated, and comfortable; and (2) it is reassurance that the patient has a patent airway and is breathing spontaneously. If in this setting the patient suddenly moves or cries out in pain in response to a surgical manipulation, it is clear that they need more local anesthesia and not more sedation. It is appropriate to provide additional sedation or analgesia for the injection of additional local anesthetic. One must proceed with caution, however. With a patient already sedated to the point of heavy snoring (perhaps even partial airway obstruction), additional medications may cause complete airway obstruction or apnea.

Before sedating a patient who has received a regional anesthetic, it must be ascertained that the block is working. If not, a sedated patient may suddenly wake up as a result of an ineffective regional block once surgical incision is made.

If a surgeon requests a "heavy MAC," a "deep MAC," or a "big MAC," they are really requesting a depth of sedation that approaches the general anesthetic side of the conscious–unconscious continuum. Although it is not appropriate to call an anesthetic a MAC when it really is a general anesthetic, it can still be termed a MAC if the patient is predominantly in the awake or lightly sedated state during the procedure. Examples of this include sedation or analgesia for a retrobulbar block in cataract surgery, local infiltration for herniorrhaphy, and local infiltration for breast biopsy. During the local anesthetic administration for each of these procedures, the anesthesiologist will often sedate the patient to the point of brief unconsciousness, knowing full well the potential need for airway support or assisted ventilation.

Plastic surgery procedures such as rhinoplasties, blepharoplasties, and liposuction are often performed under MAC anesthesia using intravenous sedation or analgesia. If anesthetic requirements are such that the patient is deeply sedated and not allowed supplemental oxygen for fear of combustion (a general anesthesia, no airway, no oxygen scenario), it is often safer to convert to general anesthesia and secure the airway with either an LMA or an endotracheal tube.

SUMMARY

Intravenous sedation is an anesthetic technique used both in and out of the operating room. Most patients will require intravenous sedation at some point in their life; their doctor may be the one administering the medications. It is therefore vital that all physicians become familiar with the basic principles and safe practice of this important technique. A fundamental concept is that a continuum exists between the conscious and unconscious states. The practitioner must be able to recognize when the patient is at risk for adverse events and take corrective action immediately. Most importantly, one must be able to establish a patent airway and provide positive-pressure ventilation if needed. This will help to ensure patient safety while making uncomfortable procedures more tolerable.

SUGGESTED READINGS

Hanley TEM, Twersky RS. Monitored anesthesia care. In: Longnecker DE, Tinker JH, Morgan GE, eds. Principles and Practice of Anesthesiology. 2nd Ed. St. Louis: Mosby 1998;2266-2286.

Hillier SC. Monitored anesthesia care. In: Barash PG, Cullen, BF, Stoelting RK, eds. Clinical Anesthesia. 3rd Ed. Philadelphia: Lippincott-Raven, 1996; 1159-1171.

Rego MMS, Watcha MF, White PF. The changing role of monitored anesthesia care in the ambulatory setting. Anesth Analg 1997;85:1020–1036.

Practice guidelines for sedation and analgesia by non-anesthesiologists. A report by the American Society of Anesthesiologists Task Force on Sedation and Analgesia by Non-Anesthesiologists. Anesthesiology 1996;84:459–471.

CHAPTER 8

Preoperative Assessment and Perioperative Management of Systemic Disease

Mary Ann Vann, MD

INTRODUCTION

Today anesthesiologists provide a wide range of services and a spectrum of care for patients, and most consider themselves to be perioperative physicians. During their first encounter with the patient, the anesthesiologist performs an evaluation, educates the patient, plans the intraoperative and postoperative care, and facilitates the optimization of any preoperative conditions. The expanded role of the anesthesiologist in the preoperative care of the surgical patient has been shown to decrease costs and improve outcomes.

The value of a preoperative meeting with the patient has been documented. An article in *JAMA* in 1963 described how a preoperative visit to the patient's hospital room the night before surgery was an effective means of relieving patient anxiety. Now that greater than 70% of patients are not admitted to the hospital before their surgical procedure, the preoperative meeting has changed location, personnel, and importance. A patient's interview with the anesthesiologist in a preoperative clinic may occur as long as 1 month before the day of surgery. The clinic anesthesiologist usually sees many patients for different surgery dates, and is often not involved in the patient's actual operating room (OR) procedure.

The financial savings of a preoperative clinic established by anesthesiologists have been illustrated at many centers, including the Cleveland Clinic and Stanford. The expanded role of the anesthesiologist has had an impact on OR scheduling and efficiency by reducing costly delays and cancellations.

The question is, "Who needs a preoperative evaluation by the anesthesiologist before the day of surgery?" Certainly there are some patients who have no medical conditions, are young, and are relatively well informed about their procedure who may be inconvenienced by having to make a trip to the preoperative clinic. For some individuals, no formal visit may be required, although they can usually request a conference with an anesthesiologist to discuss their anesthesia. These patients usually undergo a screening process to ascertain whether they meet criteria for an anesthesia assessment on the day of surgery, or whether they require special instructions before their surgery. Patient screening may be performed via a mailed questionnaire, telephone call, or online survey. Computer screening tools have been developed that can be accessed at the surgeon's office, the hospital, or home. For patients who bypass the preoperative clinic, the preoperative assessment, education, and anesthesia planning occur immediately before the OR start time.

The usual criteria for deferring the preoperative clinic visit include young age, lack of preexisting medical conditions, and transportation hardship. A common reason for a mandatory clinic visit is to conduct preoperative testing. In the past, there was an emphasis on this component of the process, and the preoperative clinics were referred to as preoperative testing. Now the names have been changed to preoperative assessment clinic or preoperative processing.

ELEMENTS OF THE PREOPERATIVE ASSESSMENT

The anesthesiologist needs to accomplish several tasks during the preoperative visit. The first and most important element of the preoperative process is the elicitation of the patient's history. This includes medical, surgical, and anesthesia histories, allergies, and a list of current medications. This history guides the rest of the preoperative visit and the plan for anesthesia care.

The patient's medical history usually begins with careful documentation of a patient's medication allergies. Certain food allergies such as soy, eggs, and shellfish, as well as latex allergy, may also be pertinent to the selection of anesthetic agents, techniques, or equipment. A list of the patient's current medications including prescription medications, over-the-counter products, herbal preparations, and dietary supplements is documented. Use of some medications may need to be altered in the preoperative period. Also, this medication list is useful in ascertaining the patient's medical history.

The patient should be questioned about current and past medical conditions. Some patients may be taking cardiac or other medications but are uncertain of their medical diagnoses. It is important to assess the patient's level of exercise tolerance. Indications of their current level of activity, such as whether an elderly patient walks, golfs, works, or only ambulates between bed and chair, give the anesthesiologist an idea of how the patient will tolerate the stress of surgery and anesthesia. A review of systems may elicit other problems or information a patient forgot to mention earlier in the interview. Likewise, the surgical history may indicate certain conditions that no longer cause the patient symptoms, but can impact the anesthetic course. Examples of these include spine surgery, cardiac surgery, and esophageal or ear, nose, and throat surgery.

A history of prior anesthetics is important. If the patient had an untoward event or bad anesthesia experience, this may influence the choice of anesthetic.

Certain conditions that are inherited may affect the patient while under anesthesia. One should inquire about a family history of anesthesia problems. These familial maladies include malignant hyperthermia (see "Malignant Hyperthermia") and atypical or deficient pseudocholinesterase. Patients will not always be able to articulate these terms, so questions are phrased in a general manner, such as "Has a blood relative ever had serious problems with a routine anesthetic?" Family members may have undergone testing for their susceptibility to these conditions. Any testing should be documented if available or researched before the OR date.

The physical examination is the next step in the preoperative assessment. This includes recording of the patient's height, weight, and vital signs. Often the patient's general appearance is indicated. This would often refer to terms such as feeble, frail, obese, or a statement of their level of mental functioning, such as alert, oriented, confused, or uncooperative. The general physical examination focuses on the heart and lungs. One finding of significance would be an undocumented murmur in children or adults that may require evaluation. The pulmonary examination is necessary to confirm the absence of rales or wheezing that may require treatment before receiving the anesthetic. It is rare for the anesthesiologist to find abnormalities on this portion of the physical examination that are not anticipated based on a good medical history. Additional areas of examination that may be useful include observation of jugulo-venous distension or auscultation of the carotid arteries for bruits.

Examination of the airway is a vital element of the preoperative physical examination. This is one means whereby the anesthesiologist can determine whether the patient may have a difficult airway and be difficult to ventilate or intubate (see Chapter 10). The airway examination begins with observation of the general appearance of the head and neck. Patients with short necks, receding chins, or beards may require special attention. The patient is asked to open their mouth, and the condition of the teeth and size of the tongue and tonsils are noted. The Mallampati airway classification requires observation of the soft palate structures and is one method used to predict the difficulty of laryngoscopic visualization of glottic structures. This classification system grades the view of the soft palate as I–IV, with class I indicating all of the soft palate and uvula are seen, and class IV indicating no soft palate is visible. The extent of mouth opening is important. Fixed limitations of jaw mobility may not allow introduction of airway devices into the mouth.

An examination of the chin and neck is also performed. The anesthesiologist will determine neck mobility in flexion and extension, the presence of neck masses or scars, and whether there is any deviation of the trachea from the midline. Also, depth of the mandible and distance from the chin to the hyoid bone should be noted.

The airway examination is performed on all patients, regardless of the planned anesthesia technique, as the ability to control the airway in an emergency is vital in all cases.

The successful placement of central neuraxis blocks (spinals or epidurals) requires the identification of landmarks. Examination of the back in the area of the planned block can give an indication of the likelihood of success. Other peripheral blocks need to be placed in areas that are free of infection. The presence of existing neurologic deficits in the patient intended to undergo a regional technique should be documented. Finally, a general assessment of intravenous access sites is useful in identifying patients in whom catheter placement may be difficult.

After completion of the history and physical examination, the anesthesiologist can decide which, if any, testing or consultation is necessary.

However, patient status alone will not determine which tests are needed; the extent of the scheduled surgical procedure also needs to be considered. Specifically, it is the invasiveness and the potential for blood loss during the surgery that guides the ordering of testing or referrals. There is a large difference in physiologic impact between a cataract procedure and a vascular procedure in the same patient.

The amount of preoperative testing has been significantly reduced during the last decade. This is true even though sicker patients with serious comorbid conditions more frequently undergo surgery today. In the past, all surgical patients underwent a panel of preoperative tests. However, it was found that routine screening with urinalysis, complete blood cell count, and chest x-ray provided little useful information that altered patient care. In fact, this testing caused harm to patients related to the workup of false-positive results.

The most frequently ordered test is the electrocardiogram (ECG). Similar studies on routine ECGs in patients have shown that they are only useful screening tools in patients at risk for cardiac disease. This group includes those with preexisting conditions, such as diabetes or hypertension, or patients in certain age groups. Many consider the groups at risk to be men older than 45 years of age, and women older than 55 years.

The most sensible rationale for preoperative testing comes from the use of algorithms or tables that consider the patient's age and physical status as well as the complexity of the surgical procedure. Routine tests, such as ECGs, that were obtained as long as 1 year before surgery are acceptable to meet preoperative testing requirements if there has been no interval change in the patient's medical condition.

Consultations are obtained when the patient's current physical status is unstable or uncontrolled, or there is not enough information to determine the patient's risk for anesthesia. The patient is usually referred to a cardiologist or internist; often this is a practitioner already familiar with the patient. This physician is expected to provide a precise medical diagnosis, clarify the extent of the patient's disease, and optimize their medical condition. Often the consultant will perform additional testing such as a stress test, echocardiogram, or pulmonary function tests. They may alter the patient's medical therapy, adding or changing the antihypertensive or antianginal medications or brondilators. The introduction of preoperative clinics run by anesthesiologists has reduced the visits to consultants by only referring those patients who will benefit from the testing or changes in therapy. Previously, surgeons who were unsure of the patient's suitability for surgery or anesthesia would refer all of their patients with certain diagnoses to consultants for clearance. Only the anesthesiologist performing the procedure can clear a patient for that anesthetic, and then only after obtaining all the appropriate information.

A significant task of the anesthesiologist is to provide the patient with preoperative education. This duty has gained importance because patients are now managing themselves at home before the surgery, and responsibility for proper preparation is placed outside of the hospital realm. During this portion of the preoperative visit, the anesthesiologist can allay the patient's concerns and facilitate the recovery process. The first step in education is the description of anesthesia techniques, so a patient knows what to expect, and can ask specific questions. For some surgical procedures, all anesthesia types, including monitored anesthesia care (MAC), regional, and general, may be suitable. In the discussion of any anesthetic, risks and alternatives are mentioned. Often the anesthesia is more risky or complicated than the surgical procedure. Distinctions among techniques that may influence the patient's preference for anesthesia include level of awareness during the procedure, risk of complications such as nausea and vomiting or headache, and limitations such as a return to work or childcare. The anesthesiologist should discuss all these elements to meet the requirements for informed consent. Any patient directives and goals of treatment for patients with chronic or terminal illness should also be noted at this time.

Finally the anesthesiologist provides the patient with preoperative instructions. These include the limits on eating or drinking before surgery. Nil per os (NPO) guidelines have been liberalized in the last several years so that certain patients may drink clear liquids on the day of surgery, usually up to 2 or 3 hours before the surgical time. However, patients who do not follow NPO guidelines are a major cause of OR delays or cancellations. Patients are instructed as to which medications they should take on the day of surgery, or discontinue some time before their OR date. For example, most cardiac medications are administered on the day of surgery, whereas drugs with anti-coagulant effects need to be discontinued up to 2 weeks before the surgery.

Once the preoperative evaluation, testing, and consultations (if necessary) are completed, the patient is assigned an American Society of Anesthesiologists (ASA) physical status. Often this occurs on the day of surgery, as some of the information is not available before then. The risks of anesthesia for a patient can be most accurately predicted on the basis of the physical status rather than any individual characteristic such as age. In some office and outpatient facilities, patient eligibility is determined solely by physical status. The assignment of physical status classification is independent of the proposed surgical procedure.

The ASA classification ranges from physical status I through V:

ASA I—Healthy patient, no preexisting disease

ASA II—Patient with mild systemic disease that does not limit activity (examples: hypertension, smoking, diabetes without complications)

ASA III—Severe systemic disease that limits activity but is not incapacitating (examples: stable angina, myocardial infarction 1–6 months old)

ASA IV—Incapacitating systemic disease, which is a constant threat to life (examples: congestive heart failure, unstable angina)

ASA V—Moribund patient, unlikely to survive 24 hours

The suffix "E" is added to the physical status for patients undergoing emergency surgery.

PERIOPERATIVE MANAGEMENT OF SYSTEMIC DISEASE

Often, plans for the OR and postoperative management of the patient with systemic disease begin during the preoperative visit. This care plan continues as the patient arrives, is prepared for the OR in the holding area, goes into the OR where anesthesia is induced, and is transferred to the recovery area. In this section, we will point out the special issues in management of the patient with different systemic disease states.

Cardiac

Cardiovascular diseases are a major risk factor for patients undergoing anesthesia. The American Heart Association and American College of Cardiology have published "Guidelines on the Perioperative Cardiovascular Evaluation for Non-Cardiac Surgery." These guidelines are useful in determining the extent of preoperative evaluation necessary for patients based on their disease states and extent of the surgical procedure. The highest risk patients are those with congestive heart failure, severe aortic stenosis, unstable angina, recent myocardial infarction (less than 1 month previous), and serious arrhythmias. These conditions warrant preoperative cardiac consultation before all but the most minor surgical procedures. Cardiac evaluation usually involves stress testing or an echocardiogram, possibly even cardiac catheterization for patients who are candidates for cardiac surgical repair. Often these cardiac patients require optimization of their medical regimen before the OR visit.

At the time of surgery, the anesthesiologist's goals include maintenance of stable vital signs and reduction of the stress of surgery. The use of β-blockers, regional anesthesia, and invasive monitoring may facilitate the achievement of these goals. A postoperative stay in the intensive care unit (ICU) is often required. An increased risk of cardiac events continues for up to 72 hours after the procedure.

Intermediate predictors of cardiac risk include mild angina, prior myocardial infarction (by history or Q waves on the ECG), compensated or prior congestive heart failure, or diabetes. If patients with these conditions are undergoing minor surgery, no further workup is necessary, and they can usually be managed using standard monitoring. For major procedures such as vascular surgery, they should receive a thorough evaluation and medical optimization, and they may require invasive monitoring and postoperative cardiac monitoring (e.g., telemetry) or ICU. All cardiac patients are advised to continue their medications in the preoperative and perioperative periods.

Respiratory

The predominant respiratory diseases affecting anesthesia management are bronchospastic conditions. Both asthma and chronic obstructive pulmonary disease (COPD) may be exacerbated by instrumentation of the airway during general anesthesia. These patients need optimization of their pulmonary condition preoperatively. Sometimes this requires addition of medications including steroids. Intraoperatively the anesthesiologist may attempt to avoid intubation by choosing a sedation or regional technique, or using a face mask or laryngeal mask airway (LMA) rather than an endotracheal tube. Postoperative ventilation is required in some patients with severe COPD or continued wheezing, but it is often preferable to remove the endotracheal tube at the end of the operation to eliminate the bronchospastic stimulus.

Smokers are asked to decrease or stop their use of cigarettes. These patients may also wheeze when intubated, and they have a higher risk of atelectasis because of secretions, and more postoperative coughing.

Patients with upper respiratory infections were once considered unsuitable for general anesthesia. Today such patients may receive general anesthesia, if they have a benign pulmonary examination and normal temperature and are undergoing a relatively brief procedure. These patients, however, may have an increased risk of pulmonary complication from atelectasis.

Gastrointestinal and Hepatic

During the review of systems, all patients should be asked about a history of gastroesophageal reflux. The frequency and timing of symptoms is important. A patient experiencing reflux only once a month after consuming a spicy meal may be treated differently from someone who cannot lie flat at night without experiencing symptoms or has radiographic or endoscopic proof of hiatal hernia or reflux. A patient with significant reflux is at risk for pulmonary aspiration. These patients should receive preoperative antacids, and they require a rapid sequence induction of general anesthesia.

Patients with liver disease are at risk for complications when the liver has decreased metabolic or synthetic function. Preoperative testing should include liver enzymes as well as prothrombin time (PT) and albumin to assess the liver's synthetic capabilities. Drug doses are usually altered in these patients owing to the abnormal levels of protein binding and clearance. The anesthesiologist also needs to consider anatomic problems, such as ascites, which may impact patient positioning, and esophageal varicosities, which may be disrupted during placement of a nasogastric tube or transesophageal echocardiography (TEE) probe. These patients often need invasive monitoring to assess their intravascular volume status. The increased risk of bleeding as a result of elevated PT or low platelets may not allow administration of central neuraxis blocks. Postoperatively, these patients may be slow to emerge from anesthesia, and may require more than usual postoperative care.

Endocrine

Diabetes is a frequently encountered comorbid condition. The preoperative assessment should delineate the presence of diabetic complications and end-organ damage. The patient needs good control of blood sugars perioperatively or they may suffer poor wound healing and infections.

Blood sugars usually rise during and after surgery and anesthesia as a result of the release of stress hormones. Oral hypoglycemic agents are usually withheld on the day of surgery. The insulin-dependent diabetic patient should be scheduled for surgery early in the day, which allows optimum management. Insulin needs to be continued to avoid hyperglycemia. Today, because 70% of surgery is performed on outpatients, elaborate schedules rather than basal requirements for insulin dosage need to be instituted in the perioperative period as the patient may be returning home to regular meals shortly after surgery. This often requires the involvement of the endocrinologist. Blood sugars are usually checked before and after surgery by glucometer or a laboratory sample. Anesthesia techniques that minimize the stress response and postoperative complications such as nausea and vomiting are preferable.

Patients receiving chronic steroid therapy need to continue supplementation during the perioperative period. For minor procedures, continuation of the usual oral medication dose is usually sufficient. For those undergoing major surgery, a "stress dose" of intravenous steroids is usually administered.

Central Nervous System

Patients who have a seizure disorder or Parkinson's disease need to continue their medications during the perioperative period. Certain anesthesia agents may decrease the seizure threshold, although other drugs, such as benzodiazepines, raise it. Parkinson's disease patients may have difficulty breathing postoperatively if they become weak or rigid as a result of decreased blood levels of their anti-Parkinsonian medications.

The patient with cerebrovascular disease is at risk for a perioperative central nervous system event. The patient with transient ischemic attacks or past history of cerebrovascular accident may experience a stroke if their anticoagulant medication is suddenly discontinued, especially during the period of hypercoagulability that may occur during and after surgery. Blood pressure in these patients needs to be tightly controlled, which may necessitate monitoring with an arterial catheter. In the patient with carotid artery stenosis, complications of catheter placement in the internal jugular vein may compromise cerebral blood flow.

Myasthenia gravis patients should not receive muscle relaxants. These patients also may be weak after the anesthetic and may require postoperative ventilation.

Hematologic

The patient with abnormal coagulation needs special consideration. These conditions arise from acquired and inherited abnormalities, as well as from medical therapy. There are several different types of anticoagulant medication available today. For some patients, medications can just be discontinued. However, other medications or conditions may require reversal of the anticoagulant effects with fresh-frozen plasma (FFP), clotting factors, or desmopressin (DDAVP) preoperatively. It takes up to 2 weeks for the effects of anti-platelet agents to resolve. Anticoagulants such as warfarin or enoxaparin (Lovenox) may require the administration of vitamin K or FFP to reverse their effects. Patients who need continuation of their anticoagulant therapy, such as patients with artificial heart valves, are usually admitted to the hospital before surgery and placed on a heparin infusion, which is discontinued only 4 to 6 hours before the surgical procedure.

Patients taking anticoagulants usually have coagulation studies (PT and partial thromboplastin time) drawn during the preoperative visit and on the day of surgery. Central neuraxis blocks are avoided in patients at risk of bleeding owing to anticoagulant therapy or abnormal or deficient platelets, because there is a risk of epidural hematoma.

The anesthesiologist may be responsible for assessing the need for blood products preoperatively and intraoperatively, and for ordering them as well. In addition, the anesthesiologist needs to ascertain the availability of compatible blood before starting a case in which the need for transfusion is likely.

Renal

Patients with renal failure may come to the OR for procedures related to their condition (e.g., creation of an arteriovenous fistula or renal transplantation) or for any other operation. The technique and schedule for dialysis should be documented, and electrolytes checked as close to the surgical time as possible. For most patients, it is best to have dialysis immediately before coming to the OR, so that their fluid balance and electrolytes are optimal at the time of surgery. The effects of certain drugs may be prolonged, whereas others are avoided entirely or the doses are reduced. Rarely, some patients require dialysis postoperatively to remove excess drugs or fluids administered during the operation.

Obesity

Obese patients experience more perioperative complications than do those of normal weight. One of the main considerations in the obese patient is the airway, as their body habitus may make it difficult to ventilate or intubate. These patients benefit from proper sniffing position achieved by placing folded blankets under the head and shoulders to facilitate intubation. They may experience problems with ventilation during and after surgery and are at risk of atelectasis.

A condition frequently encountered in obese patients is sleep apnea, both obstructive and central forms, often undiagnosed and therefore untreated. These patients are at risk for apnea after their operation because of the effects of anesthesia and narcotics used for pain management. This risk of apnea may influence the postoperative disposition of the obese patient, who may require admission to the hospital for observation after general anesthesia.

Malignant Hyperthermia

Malignant hyperthermia (MH) is an inherited condition that causes intra-cellular hypermetabolism in skeletal muscle in response to potent inhala-tion agents or succinylcholine. When a family or personal history of MH is discovered during the preoperative assessment, a plan for management needs to be instituted and discussed with the surgeon and patient. Alterna-tives to general anesthesia are recommended for these patients when appro-priate. If general anesthesia is necessary, the OR must be prepared and trig-gering agents avoided in these patients. Treatment modalities need to be readily available for these patients, including dantrolene, which can stop the hypermetabolic process, and cold intravenous fluids. After completion of surgery, MH can still occur several hours later. However, some patients are discharged to home after several hours of observation in the postanes-thesia care unit if they understand their condition and have the ability to quickly return to a hospital.

SUMMARY

Preoperative assessment is vital to the care of the patient receiving all types of anesthesia. Important elements of the preoperative assessment include the patient interview and examination, which guides the anesthesiologist in ordering tests or consultations, patient education and informed consent, and preparation and planning for the OR anesthesia management.

SUGGESTED READINGS

Guidelines for perioperative cardiovascular evaluation for noncardiac surgery. Report of the American College of Cardiology/American Heart Association Task Force on Practice Guidelines. J Am Coll Cardiol 1996;27:910–948.

Roizen MF. Preoperative evaluation. In: Miller RD, ed. Anesthesia, vol 1, 5th Ed. Philadelphia: Churchill Livingstone, 2000:824–883.

CHAPTER 9

Intravenous Access and Perioperative Fluid Management

Selina A. Long, MD

THE NECESSITY OF INTRAVENOUS ACCESS

Patients undergoing all but the most minor or atraumatic of surgical procedures require intravenous (IV) access for anesthetic drug administration as well as for fluid replacement. Fluids may be lost either as: insensible losses (evaporative), accounting for 800 to 1000 mL/day, or replacement losses (such as emesis, fistula drainage, burns, open weeping wounds, ascites, dehydrating preoperative bowel preparations, diuretic use, hemorrhage, and third-space loss). Because a significant portion of body weight is water and water rapidly equilibrates across membranes, intravascular losses may represent but a small portion of the total body water deficit (Figs. 9-1 and 9-2).

INTRAVENOUS CATHETER INSERTION

The large hand veins and the cephalic, basilic, and antecubital arm veins are the preferred sites for perioperative IV access because they provide the shortest route to the central circulation, are less frequently interrupted by the surgical site (although this needs to be considered on a case-by-case basis as in an axillary lymph node dissection), and are usually readily available to the anesthesiologist in the operating room (OR). One should

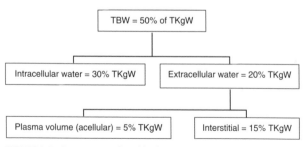

FIGURE 9-1. Composition of total body water (TBW). TKgW, total kilogram weight.

Plasma volume	+	Cellular components of blood	=	Whole blood
5% of TKgW		2.5% of TKgW		7.5% of TKgW

FIGURE 9-2. Composition of blood.

avoid using leg veins because of their lack of proximity to the anesthesiologist in the OR and their increased risk for thrombosis. The hands and arms are inspected for possible sites, looking for the longest and straightest vein possible.

Gloves must be worn to be in compliance with universal precautions, and it is most efficient if all equipment is assembled before starting the procedure. After application of a tourniquet proximal to the site, the anesthesiologist preps the skin with 70% to 90% isopropyl alcohol and allows it to dry. A small subcutaneous skin wheal of 0.5% to 1.0% lidocaine (via a 25-gauge or smaller needle) is raised to minimize the pain of IV insertion. In case of patient discomfort or agitation, more local anesthetic, gentle reassurance, or even sedation may be helpful. An IV cannula is inserted into the vein with slight backward tension on the skin for stability. As dark venous blood returns into the hub of the cannula, the catheter itself is advanced into the venous lumen and the stylet is retracted. The hub is connected to IV tubing that has been filled with fluid and had all air removed from it. Any spillage is cleaned up with sterile gauze. A sterile dressing is applied, and the tubing is secured to the skin with tape.

Patency is assured by opening the roller clamp of the IV tubing and assessing the flow rate. If a hematoma forms during an attempt, the tourniquet should be released, the catheter removed, and direct pressure immediately applied over the puncture site. Complications of IV access placement include thrombosis, phlebitis, drug or fluid extravasation (with the potential for tissue sloughing), and inadvertent intra-arterial puncture.

Although the caliber of an IV catheter is less of a concern outside the OR, during surgery the speed of drug administration and the replacement of acute blood loss are of critical importance, and therefore the diameter and length of the venous catheter matter significantly. In general, large-diameter, short catheters allow greater flow than small-diameter, long catheters. As a rule of thumb, for all but the most minor of surgeries (e.g., minor dermatologic excision), the patient should have an 18-gauge or 20-gauge catheter for access. For operations that may involve greater fluid shifts or blood losses (e.g., thoracotomy), one should consider placing one or two large-caliber (16-gauge or 14-gauge) catheters. In most cases IV access is established preoperatively because after the induction of anesthesia, the anesthesiologist may well be busy with other maneuvers such as intubation, positioning, and maintaining hemodynamic stability.

INTRAVENOUS SOLUTIONS

Choosing the appropriate IV solution is dependent on its intended purpose: will it be replacing insensible losses (in which case a hypotonic solution with respect to sodium might be preferable) or fistula drainage (perhaps a colloid instead) or acute intraoperative blood loss (then maybe isotonic crystalloid or colloid)? In actuality, surgical patients lose several different kinds of fluids concurrently. Frequently we administer a balanced technique based on the estimated or measured loss of each component. For this reason knowledge of the composition of the different IV solutions is helpful (Table 9-1).

Crystalloid solutions contain low molecular weight ions in water, with or without glucose. Colloid solutions contain higher molecular weight substances such as proteins and large polysaccharide polymers (e.g., 5% albumin and 6% hetastarch). Colloid solutions maintain plasma oncotic pressure better than crystalloid solutions because they remain in the intravascular space for 3 to 6 hours (compared with 30 minutes for the rapidly equilibrating crystalloid solutions).

Table 9-1. Composition of Crystalloid and Colloid Solutions

Solution	Tonicity (mOsm/L)[a]	NA+ (meq/L)	Cl- (meq/L)	K+ (meq/L)	Ca2+ (meq/L)	Mg2+ (meq/L)	Glucose (G/L)	Lactate (meq/L)
5% Dextrose in water (D^5w)	Hypotonic (253)	0	0	0	0	0	50	0
Normal Saline (NS)	Isotonic (308)	154	154					
D_5 ¼ NS	Isotonic (355)	38.5	38.5				50	
D_5 ½ NS	Hypertonic (432)	77	77				50	
D_5NS	Hypertonic (586)	154	154				50	
Lactated Ringer's (LR)	Isotonic (273)	130	109	4	3			28
6D_5LR	Hypertonic (525)	130	109	4	3		50	28
6% Hetastarch (in 9% NS)	Isotonic (308)	154	154					
5% Albumin	Isotonic (300)	145	145					

[a] Compared with plasma at 300 mOsm/L.

FLUID REPLACEMENT

Perioperative fluid management begins with the assessment of the patient's intravascular volume status guided by the knowledge of the extent of the surgical procedure. Preexisting intravascular volume depletion, as evidenced by dry mucous membranes, decreased urine output, tachycardia, hypotension, or clouded sensorium, should be corrected preoperatively in all but the most immediately life-threatening situations. In the presence of hypovolemia the anesthesiologist must modify the plan for induction of anesthesia, as anesthetic agents and positive-pressure ventilation frequently cause vasodilation, myocardial depression, and impaired venous return resulting in hypotension and even cardiovascular collapse.

Perioperative fluid therapy is guided by replacement of the following:

1. Fluid deficit. This primarily consists of the nil per os (NPO) deficit caused by patient fasting.

   NPO deficit = hourly maintenance rate x (number of hours NPO)

   Hourly maintenance rates based on body weights are calculated as follows:

   For the first 10 kg (0 to 10 kg): 4 mL/kg
   For the next 10 kg (11 to 20 kg): 2 mL/kg
   For all subsequent kilograms (>21 kg): 1 mL/kg

   For example, a 78-kg man is NPO for 13 hours. His NPO deficit is:
   10 x 4 mL for the first 10 kg = 40 mL
   10 x 2 mL for the next 10 kg = 20 mL
   58 x 1 mL for the remaining kilograms = 58 mL
   Total = 118 mL/h for maintenance
   118 mL/h x 13 hours = 1534 mL NPO deficit

   One should add other sources of preoperative fluid losses such as vomiting, diarrhea, or increased insensible losses owing to fever to the NPO deficit to arrive at the total fluid deficit. Half of the calculated fluid deficit usually is repleted preoperatively with the remaining half repleted during the first 2 to 3 intraoperative hours concurrent with ongoing intraoperative losses.

2. Intraoperative fluid loss. Surgical trauma leads to extravasation of fluid to a nonfunctioning or sequestered edema space commonly referred to as the third space (the first and second spaces being the intracellular and extracellular spaces) and to evaporative fluid losses based on the duration and size of the surgical exposure. One should consider the following as guidelines for the fluid replacement based on the degree of surgical trauma:

   Minimal trauma (e.g., herniorrhaphy): 0 to 2 mL/kg per hour
   Moderate trauma (e.g., open cholecystectomy): 2 to 4 mL/kg per hour
   Severe trauma (e.g., pancreatectomy): 4 to 8 mL/kg per hour

3. Blood loss. As mentioned above, crystalloid solutions rapidly equilibrate with the extravascular fluid volume, and only one third of the

volume originally administered IV remains there for any length of time. We therefore replace each milliliter of blood loss with 3 mL of an isotonic balanced salt solution such as Ringer's lactate.

While these replacements are ongoing, continuous monitoring of heart rate, blood pressure, and urine output (ideally 0.5 to 1.0 mL/kg per hour) should guide further fluid administration. The usual physiologic response to hypovolemia in the conscious person is vasoconstriction and tachycardia, which compensate and mask underlying intravascular volume depletion until 10% to 20% of the total blood volume has been lost. Anesthesia frequently blunts or completely ablates these physiologic responses, thereby accentuating the clinical response to volume losses, making estimations of intravascular volumes more complex.

ESTIMATED BLOOD LOSS

Monitoring intraoperative blood loss is another critical role of the anesthesiologist. This is based on making estimates of blood lost to suction canisters, soaked sponges, surgical drapes, and the floor. Serial hematocrit (Hct) measurements may be of some value but may overestimate or underestimate blood loss if the concurrent crystalloid infusion is overly generous or inadequate. One method of estimating allowable blood loss is as follows:

$$\text{maximal allowable blood loss (MABL)} =$$

$$\frac{\text{estimated blood volume (EBV)} \times (\text{starting Hct} - \text{lowest acceptable Hct})}{\text{average Hct during blood loss}}$$

Example: Consider a 70-kg man with a starting Hct of 46% and that you are willing to allow the Hct to drop to 25% before administering blood. How much blood loss is required to reduce the Hct to 25%? (assume 70 mL blood/kg)

$$\text{MABL} = \frac{(70 \text{ mL/kg} \times 70 \text{ kg}) \times (0.46 - 0.25)}{(0.46 + 0.25)} = 2898 \text{ mL}$$

TRANSFUSION THERAPY

When ongoing blood loss threatens organ function by decreasing the oxygen-carrying capacity of the blood, transfusion needs to be considered. One unit of packed red blood cells (PRBCs) will generally increase the patient's Hct by 3 points. Donor blood must be fully cross-matched to the patient's blood to avoid life-threatening antigen-antibody reactions. The most severe reactions occur with ABO and Rh antigen incompatibility. These antigens are present on the red cell surface and they will cross-react with antibodies present in noncompatible serum.

For example, a patient who is type A will produce anti-B antibodies in his serum and thus should not receive type B cells in a transfusion. A simple

Table 9-2.   Blood Groups and Their Compatibilities

Blood Group	Serum Antibodies	Prevalence in Population	Generally May Receive This Type of Blood
A	Anti-B	45%	A, O
B	Anti-A	8%	B, O
AB	None	4%	AB, O, A, B
O	Anti-A, Anti-B	42%	O

rule of thumb is that O is the universal donor and AB the universal recipient (assuming Rh and other cross-matching results are negative) (Table 9-2).

Finally, for all but the shortest cases, all crystalloid, colloid, and cold-stored blood should be warmed before administration to prevent hypothermia. This can be achieved through various heat-exchanging IV tubing systems. Extreme care must be taken when using pressurized IV fluid setups to vent all air before administration so as to avoid potentially massive air embolization, which could be fatal.

SUMMARY

The anesthesiologist must evaluate the surgical patient's preoperative fluid status and then obtain appropriate IV access. Perioperative fluid management includes the correction of preexisting fluid deficits and the replacement of intraoperative fluid losses. Crystalloid solutions are administered most frequently; however, colloid-containing fluids and blood products may be required in some instances. The thoughtful evaluation and treatment of the patient's volume status is a major concern of the anesthesiologist and is necessary to assure hemodynamic stability in the perioperative period.

SUGGESTED READINGS

Morgan EC, Mikhail MS. Clinical Anesthesiology. East Norwalk, CT: Appleton & Lang, 1992:477–491.

Stoelting RK, Miller RD. Basics of Anesthesia. 2nd Ed. New York: Churchill Livingstone, 1989:245–249.

CHAPTER 10

Airway Management and Ventilation

Robert I. Cohen, MD

This chapter contains information on airway assessment and management. This is one of the most basic and important skill sets learned by every physician in training. Loss of the airway and ventilation may result in brain damage or death in as quickly as 4 to 6 minutes. Drugs used for sedation, analgesia, or anesthesia are known to produce the potential for airway compromise and respiratory arrest. Whether induced by medication, trauma, or disease, alteration in level of consciousness may necessitate endotracheal intubation and delivery of mechanical ventilation. This chapter will also describe how to identify by history and physical examination which patients may be difficult to intubate and how to manage these cases.

FIRST STEPS TO AIRWAY ASSESSMENT AND MANAGEMENT

Before any procedure in which sedation, analgesia, or anesthesia will be used, careful evaluation of the patient and assuring the availability of airway equipment is important. Drugs that produce sedation and analgesia are potent depressors of the ventilatory center and may produce apnea by direct central nervous system inhibition, or by producing such profound sedation that the muscle tone necessary to maintain an open airway is lost. Readiness to open and maintain the airway begins in the operating room with a complete check of the anesthesia equipment at the start of every day, and a modified check is repeated before starting every case.

HISTORY

The first step in making sure that it will not be difficult to intubate a patient or to provide positive-pressure ventilation by mask is to take a good airway history. Some patients will report prior problems with anesthesia. For example, sore throat, hoarse voice, dental injury, or jaw pain after surgery with general anesthesia may hint that airway anatomy is altered and that the anesthesiologist had difficulty providing positive-pressure ventilation by mask or with intubation. Review the anesthesia record. Patients with sleep apnea, morbid obesity, and history of prior airway trauma or airway surgery are at increased risk. Patients with head and neck tumor or infection (such as peritonsillar abscess) may have abnormal airway anatomy and are at increased risk for loss of airway control, which could result in brain injury or death.

ASSESSMENT FOR POSSIBLE DIFFICULT AIRWAY ANATOMY: PHYSICAL EXAMINATION

The airway examination is likely to identify patients at increased risk even if the history does not. Jonathan Benumof has popularized the use of 11 criteria. There are four observations about dentition, two for the mouth and pharynx, two for the chin, and three for the neck. The more of these anatomic criteria that vary from the normal, or the greater the variation of any one criterion, the greater the chance of difficulty.

Teeth

First, note the presence and size of teeth and second, the distance between upper and lower incisors in centimeters or fingerbreadths when the jaw is maximally opened. Exceptionally long incisors may limit the view to the posterior pharynx and may make entry of a laryngoscope blade difficult. Third, note the extent to which maxillary teeth may override the mandibular teeth and fourth, the ease with which the mandible can slide forward (prognath). Does the lower jaw move sufficiently for the lower incisors to meet the upper? If the lower teeth will prognath anteriorly with respect to the upper, and if there is a large interdental distance, this suggests jaw movement will not limit airway management.

Dental and oral injuries are among the most common complications during anesthesia. Thus it is important to determine and document whether the teeth are all present, whether crowns, bridgework, or dentures are present, and whether there is evidence of poor dentition such as multiple caries or fractures, as well as loose or missing teeth. It may be better to avoid terms like "strong" or "intact" unless you actually test them with your finger during the examination, as bridgework or teeth that appear strong may in fact be quite fragile. Usually dentures are removed before the procedure so they will not become lost or broken, or become a foreign body that could enter or obstruct the airway. However, in some cases they can be left in if they fit tightly, as they may greatly assist in maintaining a good mask fit.

Mouth

A large oral cavity combined with a small, mobile tongue is a good combination for easy airway management. If the mouth is small, such as may occur with a narrow, high-arched palate, or the tongue is large with limited mobility, the risk of airway difficulty increases. A simple rating scale from 1 to 4 has been developed to quickly record this relationship and is often called the airway (or Mallampati) class (Fig. 10-1). The patient is asked to open the mouth wide, stick out the tongue, and extend the neck to optimize the view of the oral pharynx. Although this classification was originally made without asking the patient to phonate (say "ahh"), some airway experts suggest that whatever maneuver produces an optimal view should be used in scoring airway class. If the whole of the tonsillar pillars are visu-

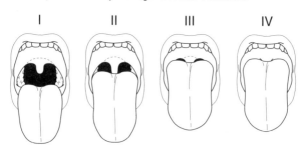

FIGURE 10-1. Mallampati class, which is determined by the volume of the oropharyngeal cavity, the tongue size, and the narrowness or arch of the palate. If the whole of the tonsillar pillars is visualized, the airway is rated class I and intubation is likely to be uncomplicated. Visualization of the uvula, but not the tonsillar pillars, represents a class II airway. Visualization of part of the uvula and soft palate is class III. If the tongue blocks the view of any structures beyond the hard palate, it is a class IV airway and is associated with increased risk of difficult intubation. Adapted with permission from Mallampati Sr, et. al. A clinical sign to predict difficulty of tracheal intubation. Can J Anaesth 33: 429-434, 1985.

alized, the airway is rated class I and intubation is likely to be uncomplicated. Visualization of the uvula, but not the tonsillar pillars, represents a class II airway. Visualization of part of the uvula and soft palate is class III. If the tongue blocks the view of any structures beyond the hard palate, it is a class IV airway and is associated with increased risk of difficult intubation. Next to presence or absence of teeth, airway (Mallampati) class is the most commonly documented airway descriptor.

Chin

The two important features of the chin for airway management include mandibular space and tissue compliance. A shorter mandible may be associated with more difficult airway management. Note that this can be more difficult to assess when the patient has a beard that conceals a receding chin. The mandibular space is bordered by the mandible anteriorly and laterally and by the hyoid posteriorly. The length between the mentum and the hyoid or the thyroid (easier to palpate, the so-called thyromental distance) is measured. Airway risk is low if the thyromental distance is three fingerbreadths or greater and the tissue compliance is high. During laryngoscopy, the laryngoscope blade displaces the soft tissues of the floor of the mouth into this region to facilitate a view of the larynx. If the thyromental distance is short or the tissue compliance is low, laryngoscopy and intubation may be difficult. Situations leading to potential difficulty include prior surgery or trauma, in which the area is fibrotic, and obesity, in which the local adipose tissue and the enlarged preepiglottic fat pad reduce airway access. Local tumor and infection also markedly reduce tissue compliance.

Neck

There are three assessment points in the neck. First, assess for full range of motion at the atlanto-occipital joint as well as the other cervical vertebrae, particularly extension and flexion. The optimal position for maintaining a patent airway is extension. That for intubation is a combination of extension at the atlanto-occipital joint and flexion at the remaining cervical vertebrae (sniffing position; Fig. 10-2). Second, painful conditions, or conditions associated with instability, such as rheumatoid arthritis, require special care, and airway control may need to be obtained by other means if movement through the full range of motion is painful or if potential instability exists. Third, if the neck is short, the larynx may take a more cephalad position and may be too anterior to visualize during laryngoscopy. If the neck is thick, as might be found in athletes who weight

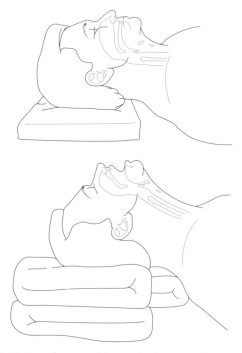

FIGURE 10-2. Alignment of the mouth, pharynx, and larynx for intubation. Note that the lower neck is well flexed whereas the upper neck is well extended (sniffing position).

train to increase the mass of the cervical musculature, it may be difficult to line up the axis of the mouth, pharynx, and larynx as is necessary to produce a line of sight needed to facilitate intubation under direct vision.

Composite scoring systems using these criteria have been developed and are effective at predicting which patients will have difficulty with airway control and intubation. An algorithm has been developed for managing patients with a difficult airway (Fig. 10-3). When there is history of prior difficult intubation or when anatomic difficulties are suggested by examination, special techniques are used to secure the airway. For example, the airway can be anesthetized with local anesthetic, the patient mildly sedated, and the airway can be intubated using a flexible fiberoptic bronchoscope designed for this purpose.

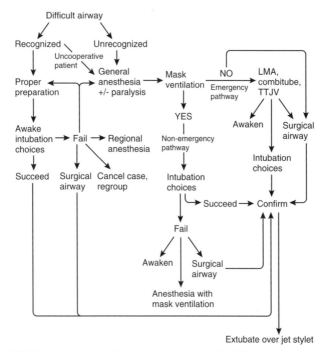

FIGURE 10-3. Algorithm for managing a patient with a difficult airway. LMA, laryngeal mask airway; TTJV, transtracheal jet ventilation. (Adapted with permission from Fisher DM, Benumof JL. Laryngeal mask airway and the ASA difficult airway algorithm. Anesthesiology 1996;84:686-699.)

MASK VENTILATION

The most fundamental skill to develop in airway management is the delivery of effective positive-pressure ventilation by means of a bag–valve–mask device (mask ventilation). The mask is soft and form-fitting, so that by pressing it firmly against the face an airtight seal is made. When air pressure in the mask increases by squeezing the inflated attached oxygen bag, air flows under pressure through the upper airway into the lungs. As the lungs expand, the chest will be observed to rise. When the bag is empty or you stop squeezing it, air from the lungs flows back out the nose and mouth into the mask. In most systems the bag is self-inflating. In the operating room a different bag–valve–mask system, built into the anesthesia machine, is used that allows exhaled gas to be recycled.

Maintaining a Good Seal

It is essential to maintain a good airtight seal between the skin of the patient's face and the mask, otherwise sufficient pressure will not develop to ensure adequate inflation of the lungs. Furthermore, it will become difficult to maintain an inflated ventilation bag if the seal is not maintained. The provider holds the mask near the top (at the 22-mm connector) between the thumb and first finger of the (usually left) hand. Pressure is applied downward (toward the face). Counterpressure is created by the fourth and fifth (if your hand is large enough) fingers hooked under the angle of the mandible and drawing it upward (toward the mask).

Leak is the most common problem. The provider must carefully apply the mask to assure a seal. If there is a good seal (no leak) and ventilation is not successful, it may be caused by airway obstruction, the next most common problem. Obstruction of the airway (usually by the tongue) is relieved by lifting the jaw, more forcefully protruding the jaw (prognathic anterior displacement), or by extending the neck. If obstruction persists, use an airway adjunct to create a passage for airflow around the tongue. If leak persists, the three-handed mask technique is recommended: while one provider holds the mask and squeezes the bag (Fig. 10-4), a second provider places the heel of each hand on either side of the mask (placing one hand over the hand of the first provider), hooks the fingertips under the mandible, and at the same time lifts the jaw (translocates anteriorly as noted above) and improves the seal by squeezing the fingers toward the palm.

Checking That Mask Ventilation Is Effective: CO_2 Detection

With each squeeze of the bag the chest should rise. A CO_2 detection device is essential for demonstrating return of air from the lungs. In the operating room this information is critical, and a capnograph (see Chapter 6) is used to provide breath-by-breath information. This device permits apnea detection within seconds. Other valuable information is obtained from the shape and size of the on-screen waveform displayed on the monitor. It is one of the most valuable monitors in the operating room.

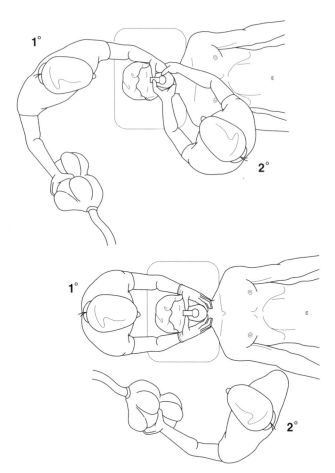

FIGURE 10-4. Leak is the most common cause of failure to ventilate effectively by mask. Until you develop the skill to do this with one hand, have an assistant place their hands over yours. Their thumbs should be on the mask over your fingers, their fingers lifting up on the jaw, again over the fingers of your left hand. Squeeze the bag so you can appreciate air flowing into the patient as you squeeze. An alternative is to use both hands to make a good seal and have the assistant squeeze the bag. (Adapted with permission from Benumof JL. Airway Management: Principles and Practice. St. Louis: Mosby Year Book, 1996. p.153)

OTHER AIRWAY EQUIPMENT

Oral Airway

The oral airway (or oral pharyngeal airway, OPA) is a curved piece of plastic that is inserted over the tongue into the pharynx. In a supine patient, in whom the tongue tends to fall backwards, closing the pharynx, the OPA provides a passage for air to flow past the otherwise obstructing tongue. To avoid trauma to the soft tissues of the mouth, a wooden tongue blade may be inserted to first press the tongue out of the way.

Nasal Airway

The nasal airway is first lubricated, then passed through the nose into the pharynx, providing a passage for air around the tongue. When passing a nasal airway, it should be directed parallel with the palate to avoid inappropriate placement. Just remember that the floor of the nose is the roof of the mouth and you will get the correct angle.

Cuffed Oropharyngeal Airway

The cuffed oropharyngeal airway (COPA), originally developed from an OPA, has a similar design and is inserted using a similar technique. Once inserted with the tip in the pharynx, an air-cuff is inflated, which optimizes its position and maximizes the relief of airway obstruction produced by the tongue. The cuff also seals off the oral and nasal pharynx so that the 22-mm connector of a bag–valve–mask device can be attached, and positive-pressure ventilation can be delivered.

Laryngeal Mask Airway

The laryngeal mask airway (LMA), like the COPA, is a cuffed device that provides sufficient seal to permit positive-pressure ventilation. The LMA is inserted into the pyriform fossa within the pharynx and is sealed when the cuff is inflated. When correctly placed and inflated, the epiglottis, which covers the larynx during swallowing, is held well away from the open larynx. The LMA is the adjunct of choice for emergency airway management when mask ventilation is not possible and laryngoscopy and intubation are unsuccessful.

When these devices are not effective, when airway control must be maintained for many hours, when mechanical ventilation is planned, or when the airway could be compromised by secretions or a foreign body, the patient will require intubation of the trachea with an endotracheal tube.

ENDOTRACHEAL INTUBATION

To prepare for intubation, the provider should make sure that basic equipment such as suction, oxygen, a bag–valve–mask device, laryngoscopes, various airway adjuncts, and various sized endotracheal tubes (ETT) are available. This is part of the precare equipment check.

Laryngoscope

The laryngoscope is designed to be held in the left hand. It is stored as two separate parts: the handle, which also serves as a battery holder, and the blade, which is used to move the tongue and soft tissues aside to reveal a view of the larynx. The laryngoscope blade attaches to the handle with the blade held parallel to the barrel of the battery case (handle), then the blade is rotated 90 degrees into a locked position that also activates the light near the tip of the blade, which illuminates the larynx.

The curved blades are called Mac or Macintosh blades; the straight blades are called Miller blades. Although both straight and curved blades expose views of the larynx for intubation, there are subtle differences in technique to obtain a good view. The straight or Miller blade is inserted deep into the oropharynx. Under direct vision, as the blade is slowly withdrawn, it will slip over the anterior larynx and come to a position at which it holds the epiglottis flat against the tongue and anterior pharynx, exposing a view of the larynx. The curved or Macintosh blade is inserted past the tongue until the tip rests at the base of the tongue in the vallecular space. Pressure is applied deep in the vallecula by the tip of the blade to evert the epiglottis and expose the larynx.

Whichever blade is used, it must not press against the teeth during laryngoscopy, or dental trauma may result. Providing sufficient lifting force in parallel with the handle, yet avoiding posterior rotation that causes the blade to press into the teeth, can be difficult to learn.

Once a view of the larynx is obtained, shift the focus of your eyes to the teeth as you introduce the ETT from the right side of the mouth. Take care that the teeth do not damage the cuff. Next, allow your focus to shift to the larynx as you observe the tip of the ETT pass into the larynx through the cords. Advance the tube until the cuff has passed through the cords 1 cm.

Document the view of the larynx obtained during laryngoscopy using a I through IV grading scale: grade I is full view of the cords; grade II is a partial view; a grade III view is obtained when the epiglottis is seen, and grade IV when it is not. Grades III and IV are considered difficult and should be noted in the patient's record.

The Endotracheal Tube

During the precare check, inspect the cuff, pilot tube, pilot balloon, and valve. Insert air to make sure pressure is maintained, and then remove all air from the cuff in preparation for intubation. A stylette, a plastic-covered malleable metal rod, may be lubricated and placed into the ETT to help maintain a more curved shape that can be more easily directed into the larynx. To prevent soft tissue trauma from a protruding stylette, bend the proximal end of the stylette over the 15-mm ETT plastic connector. Reattach the 10-mL syringe to the cuff inflation valve in readiness for intubation.

During laryngoscopy, just after the tip of the ETT is observed to pass into the larynx under direct vision, you may want to have an assistant stabilize the stylette so the ETT can be advanced over it rather than advancing them together. This may minimize trauma to tracheal mucosa. Pass the ETT cuff at least 1 cm beyond the cords for patients in the operating room. This allows less fluid to collect in the subglottic space, lessening the risk of potential aspiration at extubation. For patients who will be moved while intubated, the cuff should be closer to 2 cm beyond the cords so that the tip of the ETT lies 2 to 3 cm above the carina. This permits some outward or inward movement without allowing the ETT to either come out of the trachea or cause a mainstem bronchial intubation, respectively. However, in this case, extra care should be taken to clear oral and gastric secretions before the cuff is deflated.

Bougie

The gum-elastic bougie is a straight, semirigid, brown-colored, stylette-like device with a bent tip, often used when intubation is difficult. During laryngoscopy the provider places the tip into the larynx and—paying attention to the usual presence of vibration corresponding to the tip gently bouncing off each of the tracheal rings—gently advances it until easy advancement stops as the tip enters a mainstem bronchus. At this point, while maintaining the laryngoscope position, an assistant threads the ETT over the end of the bougie and, careful to avoid cutting the cuff on the teeth, advances the ETT over the bougie into the larynx. Maintaining the laryngoscope in position may help facilitate passage of the tip of the ETT into the larynx. When no assistant is available, it will be necessary to remove the laryngoscope and advance the ETT over the bougie without its assistance. It may be necessary to rotate the ETT 90 degrees counterclockwise for it to smoothly pass beyond the arytenoids into the larynx if the laryngoscope is removed and the tongue pushes the bougie posteriorly in the pharynx. The bougie is removed once the ETT is in place.

Connect the ETT and Check for CO_2

After insertion in the trachea, the ETT cuff is inflated with 4 to 8 mL of air, and the 15-mm connector is attached to the bag–valve device (mask removed) into which oxygen is flowing and to which the inline CO_2 detector is attached. Symmetrical right and left chest movement with the first delivered ventilation should be observed. Carbon dioxide should also be present with the first positive-pressure breath; its absence is of great concern, suggesting either incorrect placement in the esophagus or lack of CO_2 production (cardiac arrest). A mechanical ventilator is turned on at this point (or an assistant continues to squeeze the bag–valve device), while a more careful check is made of position by listening to the lung apices for equality of breath sounds.

The loss of right upper lobe sounds may be the only sign of a partial or near right mainstem bronchus intubation as this branch occurs within 1 cm of the carina. A rough confirmation of ETT cuff position can be made at this point by gently holding the pilot balloon between the thumb and forefinger of one hand while a finger on the other hand gently presses on the trachea starting at the cricoid cartilage and moving into the sternal notch, until the point is determined at which maximum variation in pilot balloon pressure is noted. At this point and from time to time during the case, the cuff pressure should be reassessed. Excessive pressure will compress the tracheal mucosa against the tracheal rings and result in mucosal necrosis and sloughing. Proper inflation will allow greater than 30 cm H_2O pressure to be applied to the ETT without hearing a leak during sustained positive-pressure ventilation.

Tape the Tube

Tape (not the cuff) is what keeps the endotracheal tube in good position. Until it is securely taped, the provider should continuously hold the ETT between the thumb and fingers near the point where it passes between the teeth. Skin overlying the maxilla and zygoma is generally preferred to skin overlying the mandible. Avoid adhesive contact with the lips to avoid tape trauma. Note the ETT position in centimeters where the tube passes the teeth or lips. Recheck that the ETT cuff is inflated enough to prevent leak when a positive-pressure ventilation is delivered, but not so much pressure that tracheal mucosal necrosis could result where the cuff compresses mucosa against the cartilaginous tracheal rings. A roll of gauze can be placed between the teeth or an OPA inserted to prevent the patient from biting and occluding the ETT during emergence from the anesthetic.

Ventilate

Continuously provide positive-pressure ventilation at a volume of 350 to 700 mL per 70 kg (5 to 10 mL/kg) and at a sufficient rate (usually 8 to 12 per minute) to maintain normal end-tidal CO_2 levels. A manometer in the breathing circuit monitors airway pressures, because injury to lung tissue, called barotrauma, can result if airway pressures are too high. Assess for good lung expansion by observing chest wall movement and listening for the presence of breath sounds in all lung fields. Frequently throughout the case, check the adequacy of ventilation and position of the ETT. All connections in the breathing circuit should be tight enough to remain attached, but not so tight that they cannot easily be disconnected by hand when required. Be alert for a sudden breathing circuit disconnect that can occur at any time, and is most likely when the patient's position changes, such as when the surgeon repositions the patient's head during a tonsillectomy. Failure to recognize disconnect could result in rapid hypoxemia, bradycardia, and cardiac arrest or, if the patient is breathing spontaneously, can rapidly result in a patient who suddenly wakes up in the middle of the case because anesthetic is no longer being delivered with each breath.

Extubation

When the case is over and the anesthetic has mostly been breathed off, and when neuromuscular blockers have been fully reversed and the patient is alert enough to protect the airway from his or her own secretions, the ETT is removed. Suction the oropharynx thoroughly. Ask the patient to lift and hold his or her head 1 inch above the pillow for 5 seconds. This demonstrates excellent motor strength, and sufficient alertness and coordination to suggest that the patient will protect the airway once extubated. (Tip: ask the patient to practice lifting his or her head at the time when you assess their airway well before giving any medication. Suggest that while they are still asleep, they will hear a voice asking them to lift their head and they should lift it just 1 inch off the pillow, hold it there for 5 seconds, then put their head back on the pillow and open their mouth. Let them know they will never remember this because it will occur near the end of surgery when they are still asleep. At emergence, you will get a crisp response to the instruction they have practiced when awake, and you will be confident that it is safe to remove the ETT at the end of the case.)

SUMMARY

Providing safe airway care is at once satisfying to the student and essential to the patient. The student is encouraged to feel accomplishment with every laryngoscopy performed as every opportunity to view airway anatomy is of value, regardless of whether the procedure was completed successfully or without assistance. Many laryngoscopies are required to learn this skill well and to recognize the wide variations of patient anatomy and matching solutions to deal with these variations. Set a goal for yourself that during your anesthesiology rotation you will acquire the skill of maintaining an open airway and delivering positive-pressure ventilation by bag–valve–mask device in an unconscious patient. This is the life-saving skill that every student should acquire during his or her time with the anesthesiologist in the operating room.

SUGGESTED READINGS

Tse JC, Rimm EB, Hussain A. Predicting difficult endotracheal intubation in surgical patients scheduled for general anesthesia: a prospective blind study. Anesth Analg 1995;81:254-258.

Rose DK, Cohen MM. The airway: problems and predictions in 18,500 patients. Can J Anaesth 1994;41(5 Pt 1):372-383.

El-Ganzouri AR, McCarthy RJ, Tuman KJ, Tanck EN, Ivankovich AD. Preoperative airway assessment: predictive value of a multivariate risk index. Anesth Analg 1996;82:1197–1204.

Fisher DM, Benumof JL. Laryngeal mask airway and the ASA difficult airway algorithm. Anesthesiology 1996;84:686–699.

CHAPTER 11

Common Intraoperative Problems and Their Management

Sheila R. Barnett, MD

Vigilance is critical during an anesthetic. The anesthesiologist must be constantly in tune with the patient and their vital signs. This chapter will address the etiology and treatment of common problems encountered during the administration of an anesthetic, many of which can rapidly deteriorate into a life-threatening situation in the absence of appropriate understanding and intervention.

Intraoperative events can be loosely divided into critical and noncritical events. Critical intraoperative problems refer to vital sign alterations and changes in oxygenation and ventilation. Examples include bradycardia, tachycardia, hypotension, hypertension, hypoxia, and hypercarbia. These events require rapid recognition and treatment to prevent complications. Many of the signs are nonspecific, so it is useful to adopt a systematic approach in dealing with critical events in the anesthetized patient.

Noncritical intraoperative events are less likely to be life threatening, but they may have a significant impact on the ability of the surgeon to complete the procedure. Examples of noncritical events include the moving patient and the inadequate regional anesthetic.

CRITICAL EVENTS

Several systems are in place to aid in the detection of a critical event, such as alarms that indicate low inspired oxygen or a disconnect monitor of the anesthesia breathing circuit. In addition the pulse oximeter is audible and alerts the anesthesiologist to changes in heart rate and saturation—the tone becomes progressively lower as the oxygen saturation drops below 98%. These are tools that alert the anesthesiologist to a problem. The following sections will discuss the etiologies of critical events and systematic approaches to intervention.

Hypoxia

Hypoxia occurs when the vital organs receive inadequate oxygen to meet tissue demand (Table 11-1). It is potentially life threatening and must be recognized and treated immediately. The tone on the pulse oximeter becomes lower as the oxygen saturation falls, and this is usually the first alteration noted by the anesthesiologist. The hypoxic patient may show

Table 11-1. Hypoxia and Hypercarbia

Hypoxia	Hypercarbia
Apnea	Apnea
Airway obstruction	Hypoventilation
Hypoventilation and ventilator failure	Bronchospasm
Esophageal intubation	Endotracheal tube obstruction
Endobronchial intubation	Increased production: sepsis, MH, thyrotoxicosis
Endotracheal tube obstruction or disconnect	Bicarbonate administration
Bronchospasm	Rebreathing: low flows
Pulmonary embolus: air, clot, fat, amniotic fluid	Rebreathing: exhausted carbon dioxide absorber
Pneumothorax	Tourniquet release
Aspiration	Laparoscopy with insufflation
Atelectasis	
Anaphylaxis	

MH, malignant hyperthermia.

nonspecific signs (e.g., confusion in the awake patient) or changes in other vital signs, such as hypercarbia, hypotension, hypertension, and tachycardia or even bradycardia (in severe cases). Hypoxia may result from numerous etiologies; therefore a practical approach is needed. Start with the patient and work back to the anesthesia machine. Patient causes of hypoxia include hypoventilation, airway obstruction, laryngospasm, endobronchial intubation, an esophageal intubation, and bronchospasm. Less common causes include pneumothorax, myocardial failure, and pulmonary embolus. Machine and circuit-related causes include circuit disconnection, circuit obstruction, and oxygen supply failure.

Always start with the patient and take action if needed. Provide the patient with 100% oxygen, either with a face mask or via the ventilator. In the ventilated patient manually ventilate with 100% oxygen while auscultating the chest to assure the presence of equal and adequate breath sounds.

In the awake patient check for upper airway obstruction, usually recognized by audible snores from the patient or rocking chest movements without any visible air movement. Changing the head position (chin lift or jaw thrust) or inserting an oral airway may be all that is needed.

Laryngospasm is a more serious cause of airway obstruction. This may be recognized by high-pitched noises during inspiration and a rapidly decreasing oxygen saturation. Laryngospasm is caused by involuntary spasm of the laryngeal musculature resulting in partial or complete closure of the vocal cords. This is commonly caused by secretions or stimulation to the posterior pharynx in the partially anesthetized patient. Immediate action is needed. First try to remove the irritating stimuli. This may be accomplished by removing an oral airway, suctioning the secretions in the posterior pharynx, or treating or relieving the painful stimuli. Although it may be possible to "break" laryngospasm by administering positive-pressure ventilation with 100% oxygen, one should be prepared to immediately intubate the patient after paralysis with a rapid-acting muscle relaxant such as succinylcholine.

Bronchospasm is the involuntary narrowing of the small airways, and is a nonspecific condition that can occur in the awake or the anesthetized patient. The key is recognition: listen to the chest for wheezing. In the awake patient wheezing may be secondary to a patient condition (such as asthma or chronic obstructive airways disease), or it may be caused by airway stimulation (e.g., aspiration). In the anesthetized patient it is often a nonspecific sign and may indicate airway irritation from the endotracheal tube or aspiration. Treat bronchospasm according to the cause.

As you listen to the chest also check the adequacy of ventilation. Is the tidal volume appropriate? Is it difficult to ventilate the patient? Are the peak airway pressures high or is the patient fighting your efforts? In the spontaneously breathing patient, inadequate tidal volumes may result in atelectasis and hypoxia. Narcotics can produce apnea and also will depress the response to hypercarbia, predisposing the patient to hypoxia. Hypoventilation is associated with hypercarbia and possibly other signs, such as tachycardia and hypertension. In a ventilated patient, set the tidal volume and respiratory rate to maintain the end-tidal carbon dioxide ($ETCO_2$) between 35 and 40 mm Hg. Depending on the patient and the surgical procedure, a tidal volume between 5 and 10 mL/kg and rate between 8 and 12 per minute are usually adequate.

Hypoxia may occur if the endotracheal tube is misplaced. Always check the tube position by auscultation and confirm the presence of $ETCO_2$ with a normal waveform. Absent breath sounds and low or absent $ETCO_2$ occur with an esophageal intubation, which requires immediate reintubation. More commonly an endobronchial intubation may occur, in which the endotracheal tube slips into a main bronchus—usually the right—and only one lung is ventilated. This can be recognized by unilateral breath sounds or wheezing and is treated by withdrawing the tube slightly.

The endotracheal tube may become kinked or obstructed. After checking for bilateral breath sounds and $ETCO_2$, trace the endotracheal tube back from the lips to the machine. Ensure the tube is not kinked or disconnected. To confirm a patent endotracheal tube one should pass a suction catheter down the tube, but this should be done cautiously, as in the lightly anesthetized patient irritation to the carina may cause coughing and bucking. Suctioning the tube will remove mucus plugs and may identify aspiration.

Oxygen supply failure is an unlikely but possible cause of hypoxia. The inspired oxygen should be checked and always maintained above 21%. The oxygen supply is checked by reading the pressure gauges at the front of the anesthesia machine, and in the event of an oxygen supply failure a distinct alarm will sound.

Less common causes of hypoxia include pneumothorax and pulmonary emboli, both of which are usually accompanied by hypotension and tachycardia. A pneumothorax in an awake patient (for instance during the placement of a central catheter) should be suspected if the patient complains of acute dyspnea and pain. In the anesthetized ventilated patient, an abrupt increase in airway pressure and absence of breath sounds accompanied by a rapid deterioration in the patient's condition with hemodynamic collapse suggest the development of a tension pneumothorax. Pulmonary emboli can be secondary to clot, air, fat, or amniotic fluid. Pulmonary emboli secondary to a clot should be suspected in the patient with acute dyspnea, chest pain, and tachycardia, especially if the patient has been immobilized for several days. Chest examination may be nonspecific with bilateral wheezes. Large emboli will cause acute cardiac failure and even arrest. Air emboli may occur whenever a vein is open to the atmosphere at a level higher than the right atrium. This may cause air to be sucked into the venous system, causing acute hypoxia and cardiovascular collapse. Air emboli are a complication of craniotomies performed in the sitting position. Fat and amniotic fluid emboli are rare causes of hypoxemia.

Hypercarbia

Hypercarbia results from either inadequate elimination, increased production, or increased absorption of carbon dioxide (Table 11-1). Physiologic consequences of hypercarbia include raised intracranial pressure (ICP), pulmonary artery hypertension, and tachycardia. Hypercarbia requires immediate investigation and treatment. As always, first ensure adequate oxygenation and ventilation. Simply increasing ventilation may be all that is required to treat hypercarbia. In the anesthetized ventilated patient adjust the ventilator to increase the respiratory rate and the tidal volume, and in the spontaneously breathing patient consider manual ventilation. The awake patient may need gentle stimulation and a reminder to breathe deeply.

Airway obstruction can impair elimination of carbon dioxide and lead to hypercarbia. This can occur from many causes, including chronic obstructive pulmonary disease, pulmonary edema, bronchospasm, and mainstem intubation.

In the spontaneously breathing patient central depression of ventilation from anesthetic agents such as the narcotics, benzodiazepines, and barbiturates may result in progressive hypercarbia. While assessing the patient determine whether the patient is narcotized or the anesthetic level is too deep. Pinpoint pupils and deep but infrequent spontaneous breaths suggest narcotic overdose. Frequently patients may respond to gentle reminders to breathe, and it is rarely necessary to reverse the effects of the opioids or benzodiazepines with naloxone (Narcan) or flumazenil.

At the end of a general anesthetic, hypercarbia may be a result of inadequate reversal of neuromuscular blockade; in this instance the patient is too weak to take adequate breaths.

During general anesthesia rebreathing of gases may result in hypercarbia. This may occur in the setting of low fresh gas flows or from the exhaustion of the carbon dioxide absorber. Rebreathing of CO_2 is indicated by an increase in the inspired CO_2 on the capnograph. Increased CO_2 absorption can occur with insufflation of the peritoneal cavity with carbon dioxide during laparoscopic procedures. Less commonly hypercarbia occurs as a result of increased CO_2 production from malignant hyperthermia (MH), sepsis, thyrotoxicosis, or sodium bicarbonate administration.

Hypotension

To prevent prolonged hypotension that can result in damage to the brain, kidneys, and heart, blood pressure (BP) should be checked at least every 5 minutes during the administration of an anesthetic (Table 11-2). BP is a function of cardiac output, systemic vascular resistance, and preload, and consequently hypotension may result from a disturbance of any of these variables. Unstable or fragile patients (or a healthy patient in whom BP manipulation will be critical) may require intra-arterial pressure monitoring for continuous beat-to-beat measurements (see Chapter 6).

During anesthesia, drug-induced hypotension is commonly encountered; consider which drugs the patient is currently taking or has recently

Table 11-2. Hypertension and Hypotension

Hypertension	Hypotension
Hypoxia	Hypoxia
Hypercarbia	Hypovolemia
Pain	Hemorrhage
Awareness, anxiety, and fear	Antihypertensive treatment
Artifact: small BP cuff	Cardiac ischemia
Epinephrine in local anesthetic solution	Tourniquet release
Drugs: pancuronium, methergine, calcium	Sympathetic blockade, e.g., spinal or epidural
Chronic hypertension	Arrhythmia
Thyroid storm, pheochromocytoma	Cardiac tamponade
Increased intracranial pressure	Tension pneumothorax
Autonomic hyperreflexia	Embolus: air, pulmonary, fat, amniotic fluid
Preeclampsia	Aortocaval compression
Renal artery stenosis	Vasovagal reaction
Bladder distension	
Alcohol withdrawal	

BP, blood pressure.

been given. Decreased systemic vascular resistance is very common in the anesthetized patient, and may be caused by certain drugs such as isoflurane, the barbiturates, propofol, and the benzodiazepines (the latter especially when combined with an opioid). Less common causes of vasodilation and hypotension include the release of histamine from drugs such as atracurium, curare, and morphine. Other signs such as flushing, urticaria, and bronchospasm as well as hypotension frequently accompany histamine release in the susceptible patient. Most anesthetic agents may also depress cardiac contractility. Narcotics are the exception and do not cause direct cardiac depression; however, opioids may indirectly depress BP by reducing sympathetic outflow. Calcium-channel blockers, β-blockers, and lidocaine are some of the cardiac medications that depress cardiac contractility.

Hypovolemia is also very common in the surgical patient, often accompanied by tachycardia. The surgical patient has usually been nil per os (NPO) for many hours before the surgery and may be sustaining a substantial ongoing fluid loss (e.g., during bowel surgery) or blood loss. Aids in the detection of hypovolemia include central venous pressure measurements and such laboratory tests as the base deficit and hematocrit. Clinical signs of hypovolemia include tachycardia, low urine output, and exaggerated declines in the BP during positive-pressure ventilation.

Spinal and epidural anesthesia predictably cause hypotension through sympathetic blockade and vasodilation, usually responsive to fluid and vasopressor treatment with ephedrine. Extremely high levels of spinal blockade — a total spinal — can result in resistant hypotension and bradycardia requiring immediate resuscitation.

Acute events such as cardiac tamponade, tension pneumothorax, and a pulmonary embolus from air, clot, fat, or amniotic fluid are all causes of abrupt and frequently catastrophic hypotension. During orthopedic surgery hypotension may be seen after the release of a tourniquet—probably secondary to active metabolites and lactic acidosis. Similarly, after release of an aortic cross-clamp in aortic aneurysm surgery there can be profound hypotension. Myocardial ischemia and failure, sepsis, and anaphylaxis are less common causes of hypotension. Inadequate venous return may occur in the sitting position, in the pregnant patient in whom the gravid uterus obstruction can cause aortocaval obstruction, and in mechanically ventilated patients with high levels of positive end-expiratory pressure.

Acute bradycardia and hypotension may occur during a vasovagal reaction. It is most common in the hypoxic patient under a light anesthetic, but it may also occur during eye surgery from traction on the globe, or during laparoscopic surgery in response to peritoneal stretch after insufflation of the abdomen. It is a vagally mediated response treated by removing the stimulus or occasionally with atropine.

In addition dysrhythmias, electrolyte imbalance (hypocalcemia, alkalosis, acidosis), and severe hypothermia below 32°C may result in depressed cardiac function and subsequent hypotension.

Once hypotension is detected, management should be immediately directed at diagnosis and treatment. As always first ensure adequate oxygenation and ventilation. Next consider likely causes using a systematic approach. Decreasing the anesthetic and administering a fluid bolus and possibly a short-acting vasopressor such as ephedrine or phenylephrine can help temporize during the evaluation. The definitive treatment will depend on the underlying cause of the hypotension.

Hypertension

There are many causes for hypertension in the anesthetized patient, and it is a nonspecific sign frequently accompanied by tachycardia (Table 11-2). First always rule out hypoxia and hypercarbia as causes of hypertension. Once adequate oxygenation and ventilation have been assured consider the differential diagnosis. Does the patient have a history of preexisting hypertension? Check whether they have received their usual medications. Rebound hypertension is seen in acute withdrawal from clonidine or β-blockers. Is the patient adequately anesthetized? Hypertension commonly occurs in response to light anesthesia, pain, anxiety, and awareness. Sympathetic stimulation during laryngoscopy and with manipulation of the endotracheal tube results in hypertension, and this may be more pronounced in the elderly and those with preexisting hypertension. Has the patient received a large amount of intravenous fluid without voiding? Bladder distension can be uncomfortable and cause hypertension. Always check the surgical field—infiltration with a local anesthetic and epinephrine solution can result in hypertension from absorption of epinephrine.

Certain drugs may cause hypertension such as pancuronium and vasopressors like ephedrine and phenylephrine. Alcohol and recreational drug withdrawal can present with hypertension and signs of sympathetic overactivity.

Some causes of hypertension are unique to the type of patient; in the pregnant or recently delivered patient the hypertension may indicate preeclampsia (see Chapter 16). Autonomic hyperreflexia may occur during minor procedures in patients with spinal cord injuries. Rarer causes of hypertension include intracranial hypertension, pheochromocytoma, and thyroid storm.

Hypertension during an anesthetic can be dangerous to the patient and requires recognition, assessment, and treatment. The treatment should be aimed at the underlying etiology. Once other causes have been ruled out, hypertension is usually treated by increasing the anesthetic depth with narcotics and volatile agents. Short-acting antihypertensive drugs such as nitroglycerin or labetalol are often used for the patient with persistent hypertension despite adequate anesthesia.

Dysrhythmias

The approach to abnormal rhythms is similar for most of them; the actual treatment depends on the underlying cause (Table 11-3). First rule out hypoxia, hypercarbia, and blood pressure abnormalities.

Sinus bradycardia (Table 11-3) may occur in response to hypoxia, especially in children and infants. In adults slow heart rates are common, especially in athletes as a result of high resting parasympathetic tone. Sinus

Table 11-3. Bradycardia and Tachycardia

Bradycardia	Tachycardia
Hypoxia	Hypoxia
Increased ICP	Hypercarbia
β-Blockers, calcium-channel blockers	Pain
Sick sinus syndrome	Hypovolemia
Vagal reflex	Hemorrhage, anemia
Intrinsic bradycardia	Epinephrine with local anesthetic solution
Total spinal	Volatile agents, e.g., isoflurane and desflurane
Hypothermia	Withdrawal of drugs: β-blockers, alcohol, narcotics
Hypothyroid	Anxiety and fear
Pacemaker failure	Awareness
Anticholinesterases	Emboli: air, fat, clot, amniotic fluid
Cardiac ischemia	Alcohol withdrawal, sepsis, MH, thyrotoxicosis, pheochromocytoma, bladder distension

ICP, intracranial pressure; MH, malignant hyperthermia.

bradycardia is usually well tolerated, and in fact it may be desirable in the patient with coronary artery disease.

Medications that cause bradycardia include opioids, β-blockers, calcium-channel blockers, and succinylcholine. In adults bradycardia from succinylcholine usually occurs only after a second dose. Sick sinus syndrome and cardiac ischemia can result in sinus bradycardia.

Vagally mediated reflexes can cause profound acute bradycardia and even asystole. Examples include hypoxia, light anesthesia, peritoneal stretch during hernia repair, insufflation of the abdomen during laparoscopy, and traction on the globe during eye surgery.

Increased ICP may be associated with hypertension and bradycardia, with treatment aimed at reducing the ICP and the systemic blood pressure. Anticholinesterase overdose is a cause of bradycardia. A high spinal or epidural anesthetic level can result in bradycardia if the cardiac accelerator fibers are blocked.

After adequate ventilation and oxygenation have been assured, treatment should be directed toward the underlying cause. Usually treatment of sinus bradycardia is reserved for symptomatic or hypotensive patients. If required, atropine or glycopyrrolate are anticholinergic drugs, which can be administered rapidly intravenously. If bradycardia is associated with severe hypotension, then a sympathomimetic agent such as ephedrine or epinephrine may be a better choice.

Sinus tachycardia (Table 11-3) is frequently a nonspecific sign often accompanied by hypertension or hypotension. There are multiple causes including light anesthesia, hypercarbia, hypoxia, hypotension, hypovolemia, hemorrhage, and certain drugs such as pancuronium and glycopyrrolate. Rarer causes include thyrotoxicosis, pheochromocytoma, and MH. Once inadequate anesthesia has been ruled out, treatment should be directed at the underlying cause. A short-acting β-blocker such as esmolol may be useful as a temporizing agent while the cause is investigated.

Ventricular dysrhythmias may reflect underlying cardiac disease, electrolyte disturbances (e.g., hypokalemia and hyperkalemia), and digoxin overdose. Ventricular ectopy may also occur with catecholamine surges—for instance with stress, pain, and anxiety. Rare causes include thyrotoxicosis, pheochromocytoma, and MH. Lidocaine is useful for treatment of most ventricular ectopy; however, the underlying cause should be sought. For more malignant ventricular arrhythmias such as pulseless ventricular tachycardia or ventricular fibrillation, immediate cardioversion followed by amiodarone administration is now recommended.

First-degree heart block tends to be benign and is characterized by prolongation of the PR interval. It is commonly observed in patients on β-blockers.

Second-degree heart block is divided into Mobitz type I and II. Type I is generally benign, and characterized by gradual lengthening of the PR interval and subsequent drop of a QRS complex after a P wave. It only requires treatment if there are associated problems such as hypotension or congestive heart failure. Mobitz type II is more serious, as it poses a real threat of progressing to complete heart block. It is characterized by an occasional dropped QRS complex after a P wave and suggests distal atrioventricular nodal disorder. Third-degree heart block or complete heart block is recognized by the absence of a coordinated P wave and QRS complex and a slow rate. Treatment for third-degree and Mobitz type II heart blocks is cardiac pacing.

Myocardial Ischemia

Myocardial ischemia occurs when there is inadequate blood supply to meet the oxygen demands of the heart, and if untreated can lead to myocardial infarction and even death. In the awake patient signs of ischemia such as chest pain or dyspnea may accompany electrocardiographic changes and allow early recognition. However, in the anesthetized patient signs of ischemia can be nonspecific, including hypotension, ventricular ectopy, and increased pulmonary artery pressure. Ischemia frequently occurs in the setting of hypertension and tachycardia, and therefore β-blockers can be used to slow the heart and decrease myocardial oxygen demand. In addition, an infusion of nitroglycerin can be used to decrease preload (decreases myocardial oxygen demand) and to produce coronary artery vasodilation (increases oxygen supply). All patients with intraoperative ischemia require further cardiac evaluation during the recovery period (see Chapter 12).

Hypothermia

Hypothermia is common in surgical patients. The cold operating room, the administration of cold fluids and gases, and the surgery itself all contribute to the development of hypothermia. All patients undergoing anesthesia should have temperature monitoring available, usually using an oropharyngeal probe in the asleep patient. Temperature measurement is important to prevent hypothermia and ongoing temperature loss. Heat loss occurs through radiation (60%), evaporation (20 %), convection to the surrounding room (15%), and conduction to a cooler surface (5%). Volatile anesthetic agents and regional anesthetics impair temperature regulation and predispose the patient to hypothermia. Hypothermia increases demands on the cardiovascular system, increasing systemic vascular resistance and myocardial work. Shivering can increase the oxygen consumption by 100% to 200%. In addition hypothermia can reduce metabolism of certain drugs, such as neuromuscular blockers, and can result in diminished tissue perfusion leading to lactic acidosis.

The best treatment for hypothermia is prevention. Keep the patient warm in the holding area, and raise the operating room temperature before entering. Active warming is best accomplished with warming blankets (such as the Bair Hugger, Augustine Medical, Inc., Eden Prairie, MN) and by warming intravenous fluids. In addition airway humidifiers can reduce evaporative heat loss.

Hyperthermia

Hyperthermia is defined as a rise in temperature at a rate of greater than 0.5°C per 15 minutes or 2°C per hour, and is usually accompanied by a hypermetabolic state. Although rare, MH is the most serious of all causes of hyperthermia, and it must be ruled out and rapidly treated with dantrolene if suspected. More common causes of temperature elevation include atelectasis, infection, and sepsis. It is unlikely that a patient will become hyperthermic from attempts to conserve temperature.

Anaphylactic and Anaphylactoid Reactions

Anaphylactic and anaphylactoid reactions are serious events that may occur very rapidly. Anaphylactic allergic reactions involve antigen binding with IgE immunoglobulins, which results in a rapid cascade of events secondary to the release of histamine, leukotrienes, and other vasoactive substances. Anaphylactoid reactions are similar but they involve non–IgE-mediated histamine release. The clinical presentations of both are similar; urticaria, flushing, wheezing, pulmonary edema, and hypotension are key features of these reactions. Rapid recognition is essential, and if suspected, immediate treatment should be given. If the patient is unstable, discontinue anesthetic agents, provide 100% oxygen, and give an intravenous fluid bolus. The treatment of choice is epinephrine, starting with a bolus of 5 to 10 μg followed by a low-dose infusion in the hypotensive patient. Additional epinephrine and vasopressor support is indicated depending on the patient's condition. Steroids and histamine antagonists such as diphenhydramine are often added.

THE NONCRITICAL EVENT

An ideal anesthetic is one that provides the patient with a positive safe experience and the surgeon with excellent surgical conditions to perform the operation. This means that although noncritical events discussed below may not threaten the life of a patient, they may adversely affect operating conditions and also distract the surgeon from the task. Similarly the patient may not remember the superb job the anesthesiologist did treating their life-threatening bradycardia, but they will probably never forget the pain they felt when the spinal wore off prematurely or the time they spent in the recovery room feeling drowsy and drugged.

"I Can't Close"

This is commonly encountered at the end of an abdominal surgery such as a colectomy or exploratory laparotomy. As the neuromuscular blocker wears off at the end of the case the abdominal muscles tighten, and it can become very difficult to close the peritoneum. This may be worsened as the anesthetic lightens and the patient attempts to breathe. Difficulty closing is more common in younger patients with strong muscles, but fortunately it is unlikely to be life threatening. There are a few options for treatment — first reassure the surgeon you are addressing the problem. The goal is to relax the patient's muscles and prevent further spontaneous movements. This may be accomplished by deepening the anesthesia with a volatile agent or by giving a bolus of a short-acting anesthetic like propofol. This may provide enough relaxation to allow the surgeon to close. If the wound is large or very tight, small doses of a short-acting neuromuscular blocker may be necessary, remembering it will soon be time to reverse the blockade.

"The Patient Is Moving"

This requires immediate attention and usually indicates inadequate anesthesia. The first step is to deepen the anesthetic. Depending on the situation, options include increasing the volatile anesthetic, giving an intravenous bolus of a hypnotic agent such as propofol or sodium thiopental, and giving additional narcotics. After deepening the anesthetic, check the neuromuscular blockade status and titrate in neuromuscular blockade as needed.

"Ouch, That Hurts" During a Regional Anesthetic

This is a bad scenario all round—the patient is in pain and usually anxious, and the surgeon will be unable to continue the operation. Do not doubt the patient—if the patient says it hurts, there is pain. If a regional technique is used, consider the timing of the placement of the block—has there been adequate time? Some regional anesthetics—especially nerve blocks such as axillary or sciatic—can take up to 45 minutes to reach full effect. If this is the case, discuss waiting or having the surgeon supplement the block with a local anesthetic infiltration. In addition one can administer intravenous sedatives and analgesics such as fentanyl and midazolam. Despite these measures, it is sometimes necessary to convert to a general anesthetic.

The Surgery Is Over, the Gases Are Off, and the Patient Is Not Responding

Always check the vital signs first—are they stable? The common causes of a slow wake-up are residual inhaled anesthetic gases and narcotics. The expired concentration of inhaled agents can be assessed by the gas analyzer—if substantial amounts are still present, continue to ventilate with 100% oxygen until they are washed out. This may take as long as 15 minutes with the more soluble gases such as isoflurane. Also check for pinpoint pupils, suggesting that a relative overdose of narcotic may be responsible. Allow the end-tidal CO_2 to rise slowly and see whether the patient breathes spontaneously. Inadequate reversal of neuromuscular blockade or prolonged blockade may be secondary to undiagnosed psuedocholinesterase deficiency or myasthenia gravis. When in doubt, always err on the side of caution, and take the patient to the recovery room with the endotracheal tube in place until awake.

SUMMARY

Vigilance is the cornerstone of anesthetic management. One must constantly be alert for the slightest changes in the patient's clinical signs and overall condition and must develop strategies to quickly assess the patient and to take appropriate action. Early management of critical events is the best way to prevent a disaster, and immediate intervention can ultimately be life-saving.

SUGGESTED READING

Hurford WE, ed. Clinical Anesthesia Procedures of the Massachusetts General Hospital. 5th Ed. Philadelphia: Lippincott-Raven, 1998.

CHAPTER 12

The Postanesthesia Care Unit and Management of Common Postoperative Problems

Samir K. Patel, MD

INTRODUCTION

For most patients recovery from anesthesia is a smooth and uneventful process after an uncomplicated operation. However, for some patients, recovery from anesthesia can be a life-threatening process best managed by prompt intervention delivered by skilled medical and nursing personnel. The postanesthesia care unit (PACU) has the challenge of simultaneously caring for patients waking up after routine surgery, patients recovering from regional anesthesia, and occasionally critically ill postoperative patients.

Although methods of general anesthesia have been available for more than 150 years, PACUs have only become common in the past 40 years. An early description came in 1863, when Florence Nightingale wrote: "It is not uncommon, in small country hospitals, to have a recess or small room leading from the operating theatre in which the patients remain until they have recovered, or at least recovered from the immediate effects of the operation."

The last two decades have seen a dramatic increase in outpatient surgery, and PACUs must now manage patients who will be going home following anesthetic recovery and not admitted to a hospital ward. The modern PACU is located close to the operating suite to allow anesthesiologists and surgeons to be close by, and to permit a rapid return of the patient to the operating room, should it be required. There is also immediate access to radiologic imaging, blood bank, blood gas analysis, and other clinical laboratory services.

MONITORING EQUIPMENT

Inasmuch as patients recently transported from the operating room are at risk of hemodynamic and airway compromise, the ability to rapidly and continually monitor patients is essential. Automated sphygmomanometers and pulse oximetry are an essential monitoring technique in the PACU. Electrocardiographic monitoring is also routinely available for all patients. The capability for direct intra-arterial blood pressure and intracranial pressure monitoring is required in those hospitals treating critically ill patients. Emergency resuscitation equipment must also be immediately available and should be located in the PACU. A fully stocked "crash cart" containing cardiopulmonary resuscitation equipment and emergency drugs should be nearby at all times, as should an airway cart consisting of oral and nasal airways, endotracheal tubes, and laryngoscopes. Self-inflating Ambu bags with positive end-expiratory pressure valves are required for mask ventilation. A fiberoptic bronchoscope should also be available.

RECOVERY FROM ANESTHESIA

After tracheal extubation, the patient is transferred from the operating room table to a stretcher. The patient may be transported from the operating room in the lateral position to reduce the risk of airway obstruction or aspiration of gastric contents from vomiting.

When the patient arrives in the PACU, the anesthesiologist gives the nurse a full report of the events during surgery. This report should include the patient's name, age, surgical procedure, medical problems, preoperative medications, allergies, anesthetic drugs and methods, fluid and blood replacement, blood loss, urinary output, gastric output, and surgical or anesthetic complications encountered.

After major surgical procedures, all patients should receive oxygen therapy via a face mask or nasal prongs. Healthy patients, after undergoing a brief minor surgical procedure, may not require oxygen therapy; this can be guided by pulse oximetry. The routine administration of oxygen in the PACU is mildly controversial in the modern PACU equipped with pulse oximeters. The nurse should be informed of any special medications, tests, or procedures that will be required in the PACU. Vital signs should be recorded at least every 15 minutes during the first postoperative hour, and more frequently in the unstable patient. Patients should also be encouraged to awaken, cough, and breathe deeply.

Discharge Considerations

Some patients may meet discharge criteria on arrival to the recovery room. All patients should be seen again by an anesthesiologist before being discharged from the PACU, and the patient's condition should be recorded as a note in the chart. Before discharge, the patient who has undergone general anesthesia should be easily arousable and oriented, have stable vital signs, and be comfortable.

POSTANESTHESIA CARE

Respiratory Complications

The major respiratory complications encountered in the PACU are airway obstruction, hypoxemia, hypercapnia, and aspiration. Prompt recognition and treatment of these life-threatening problems are crucial to good postanesthesia care. A wide variety of factors can increase the risk of airway complications, such as obesity, increased age, prolonged or emergency operations, use of high-dose opioids, and the use of thiopental in contrast to propofol for induction of anesthesia. These patients have longer PACU stays and more cardiovascular problems, and they are more likely to require admission to the intensive care unit.

AIRWAY OBSTRUCTION

The most common cause of postoperative airway obstruction is pharyngeal obstruction from a relaxed tongue in the unconscious patient. Obstruction can also occur as a result of laryngospasm or direct injury to the airway. The most effective method of dealing with pharyngeal obstruction is a combination of a backward tilt of the head with an anterior displacement of the mandible. If the obstruction is not immediately reversible, a nasal or oropharyngeal airway may be inserted. The nasal airway is often better tolerated, and an oral airway may stimulate gagging or vomiting as well as laryngospasm. For all cases of airway obstruction, if an adequate airway cannot be reestablished by these simple maneuvers, the patient must be reintubated. The insertion of a laryngeal mask airway (LMA) may be useful in certain patients and has been used to provide ventilatory support in the PACU. In the rare case in which the trachea cannot be intubated, an emergency cricothyroidotomy will provide a means for emergent oxygenation, and this is a safer procedure than an emergency tracheostomy. Prompt action is crucial in airway obstruction because the partial pressure of arterial carbon dioxide ($PaCO_2$) increases rapidly, and there is also a progressive fall in the arterial partial pressure of oxygen (PaO_2), owing to the continuous depletion of alveolar oxygen (PAO_2).

Patients with a history of obstructive sleep apnea have a higher risk of airway obstruction while sedated, and the application of continuous positive airway pressure (CPAP) by a nasal or facial mask can be particularly therapeutic in the postoperative period.

HYPOXEMIA

Hypoxemia is a common and potentially serious postoperative complication (Fig. 12-1). Hypoxemia after anesthesia and surgery can be caused by many factors, including a low inspired concentration of oxygen (FIO_2) as may be seen in a medical gas supply disruption or misconnection, hypoventilation, areas of ventilation–perfusion mismatch, and an increased intrapulmonary right-to-left shunt. Situations such as increased age, postoperative shivering, and a lowered cardiac output may worsen the degree of hypoxemia in these patients.

A low inspired concentration of oxygen ($FIO_2 < 0.21$) is a serious, but thankfully rare, cause of postoperative hypoxemia. The most common cause of postoperative hypoxemia is an increase in the right-to-left intrapulmonary shunt, which can be caused by many processes. Pulmonary atelectasis is the most common cause and is usually the result of segmental lung collapse with a loss of alveolar volume. Bronchial obstruction from secretions or blood is another cause, and is best managed by adequate humidification of the inspired gases, coughing, deep breathing, chest physical therapy, and postural drainage. An endobronchial intubation with collapse of the opposite lung is a potentially serious complication and must be avoided by ensuring the accuracy of endotracheal tube placement.

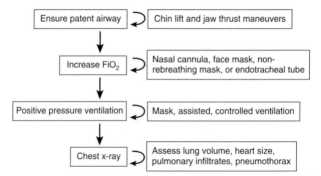

FIGURE 12-1. Initial management of hypoxemia. FiO_2, fraction of inspired oxygen.

Pneumothoraces as a cause of hypoxemia may have serious sequelae, and result in atelectasis and an increased intrapulmonary shunt. A pneumothorax usually occurs as a result of direct lung or airway injury from trauma, rib fractures, or attempts at percutaneous central venous cannulation. Those resulting from mechanical ventilation are rare unless airway pressures are particularly high. Treatment depends on the size of the pneumothorax and the patient's clinical condition, but usually requires chest tube insertion and drainage with a one-way underwater seal. A tension pneumothorax occurs when the pleural cavity fills with air, which then compresses the mediastinum and thus impairs the return of venous blood to the heart. Tension pneumothoraces are treated in the same manner, although in an emergency with hypotension there should be no delay in decompression of the chest—a 14-gauge needle must be immediately inserted in the second intercostal space in the mid-clavicular line of the chest wall to relieve the thoracic tension before formal chest-tube drainage.

Pulmonary edema may result in hypoxemia in the postoperative period and occurs most commonly within the first hour after the completion of surgery. Detection is frequently made by the presence of wheezing on auscultation of the chest. Pulmonary edema develops because of high hydrostatic pressures in the pulmonary capillaries, increased capillary permeability, or sustained reductions in the interstitial hydrostatic pressure. The latter type is seen after prolonged airway obstruction, and is often termed "negative-pressure pulmonary edema." High-pressure pulmonary edema is usually secondary to ischemic or valvular heart disease. Pulmonary edema characterized by a permeability injury is seen after a wide variety of serious clinical situations such as disseminated intravascular coagulation, shock, trauma, massive transfusion, sepsis, and anaphylaxis. This type of pulmonary edema is frequently called the adult respiratory distress syndrome, or ARDS, and is characterized by hypoxemia, diffuse pulmonary infiltrates on chest x-ray, and reduced lung compliance in the setting of adequate cardiac function. Respiratory support with oxygen and mechanical ventilation are frequently necessary while the patient receives definitive treatment. Vomiting and aspiration of gastric contents during and after anesthesia can also produce a severe permeability injury resulting in pulmonary edema and hypoxemia.

Pulmonary embolism occurring in the immediate postoperative period is a potentially fatal condition that can lead to profound hypoxemia. Patients on bed rest for prolonged periods are at an increased risk of emboli. The diagnosis is suspected in a patient with sudden pleuritic chest pain, shortness of breath, pleural effusion, or tachypnea. Right heart strain may be detected on the electrocardiogram (ECG). Massive emboli result in hypotension and pulmonary hypertension with an elevated central venous pressure, and there is a potential for right heart failure. Because the treatment of choice is anticoagulation, accurate diagnosis is important so that patients are not needlessly exposed to its inherent risks. The current standard for diagnosis is pulmonary angiography, and this is often the procedure of choice for these patients. If emboli recur or if bleeding develops, an inferior vena caval filter may be placed.

The type of anesthetic and the site of operation influence the reduction in Pao_2 seen after anesthesia and surgery. Also, postoperative shivering can result in dramatic increases in oxygen consumption.

Treatment of hypoxemia by face mask oxygen is effective in restoring the Pao_2 in many cases. The Pao_2 response to oxygen therapy is related to the degree of intrapulmonary shunt, with little effect on the Pao_2 in patients with a large shunt fraction.

CPAP by an external mask (mask or nasal CPAP) is increasingly used for treatment of patients with severe hypoxemia who have adequate carbon dioxide elimination (i.e., ventilation). Good candidates for mask or nasal CPAP are patients with severe hypoxemia requiring more than 80% oxygen to achieve a Pao_2 higher than 60 mm Hg. They must have a normal or low $Paco_2$, should not have severe respiratory distress, and must be awake and alert. Mask or nasal CPAP is most useful when the cause of hypoxemia can be quickly corrected (e.g., cardiogenic pulmonary edema) because the mask becomes uncomfortable for patients after several hours of use. Newer mask designs have improved on this problem somewhat.

HYPOVENTILATION

Hypoventilation is defined as reduced alveolar ventilation resulting in an increase in the $Paco_2$. During the postoperative period, hypoventilation occurs as a result of poor respiratory drive, poor respiratory muscle function, a high production rate of carbon dioxide, or acute or chronic lung disease.

Narcotic-induced respiratory depression can be reversed by use of narcotic antagonists. When small doses are used, these agents can reverse the narcotic-induced respiratory depression without altering pain relief; however, the duration of action of currently available antagonists is shorter than most narcotics, and the dose often has to be repeated at least once. Larger doses reverse the analgesic effects of the narcotics and result in a patient in severe pain, which can lead to increases in myocardial oxygen consumption and ischemia in patients with coronary artery disease.

Poor respiratory muscle function occurs after surgery and often contributes to hypoventilation. The site of the incision affects the ability to take a large breath, as measured by vital capacity assessment. Nearly all patients have reductions in vital capacity that is greatest on the day of surgery, and those undergoing upper abdominal surgery show the largest fall, with as much as a 60% reduction.

Failure of reversal of neuromuscular blocking agents may result in inadequate respiratory muscle function postoperatively. This can be caused by inadequate excretion of the drug (such as in renal failure) or by the presence of other drugs that accentuate neuromuscular blockade, such as gentamicin, neomycin, clindamycin, or furosemide. Hypermagnesemia also potentiates neuromuscular blockade, as does hypothermia.

Obesity, gastric dilation, tight wound dressings, and body casts also inhibit respiratory muscle function and predispose to carbon dioxide retention. A high level of carbon dioxide production from sepsis or shivering can also result in carbon dioxide retention, especially if the patient is unable to increase minute ventilation.

The vital capacity generated by the patient should be at least 10 mL/kg body weight, and the inspiratory force should be numerically greater than 20 cm H_2O. If these minimum values cannot be maintained, the patient should receive controlled mechanical ventilation until he or she is awake enough to generate adequate respiratory muscle function.

Treatment of serious respiratory failure necessitates emergency tracheal intubation. The need to perform reintubation is rare, occurring in 0.2% of approximately 13,000 patients studied in one series. Many of the cases were related to excessive anesthetic and sedative dosing, excessive fluid administration, the persistent effects of muscle relaxants, and the development of upper airway obstruction.

Circulatory Complications

Critical cardiovascular events in the PACU are the second major group of life-threatening complications for patients in this setting. The risk factors for cardiovascular complications and the ultimate outcome were evaluated by Rose and colleagues in a study of 18,380 patients after general anesthesia in Toronto. These investigators found that patients who developed hypertension or tachycardia in the PACU had more unplanned intensive care admissions and a higher mortality rate than those who did not. In contrast to respiratory events, anesthetic factors only contributed in a minor way to the development of cardiovascular problems in the PACU, whereas patient and surgical factors were more important risk factors.

HYPOTENSION

Hypotension in the recovery phase of anesthesia usually signifies decreased ventricular preload, reduced myocardial contractility, or a profound reduction in systemic vascular resistance. Decreased ventricular preload is caused by intravascular volume depletion owing to blood loss, excessive third-space fluid loss, unreplaced urinary losses, or septicemia with vasodilation and capillary leakage of fluid. Acute, massive pulmonary embolism produces hypotension by occluding the flow of blood to the left heart. Reductions in myocardial contractility occur because of continued effects of anesthetic drugs, preexisting ventricular dysfunction, or the development of a perioperative myocardial infarction. Profound reductions in systemic vascular resistance usually occur with septicemia, and they are also seen in chronic liver failure.

Prompt diagnosis and treatment are important, because prolonged hypotension can result in hypoperfusion of vital organs and subsequent ischemic injury. One must quickly assess whether the hypotension is real or an artifact of the measurement system. If the hypotension is real, ventricular preload can be increased by elevation of the patient's legs and administration of intravenous fluids. Normal saline and lactated Ringer's solution are effective and inexpensive choices. The surgical wound should be examined for evidence of rapid blood loss, and a hemoglobin level checked. If hypotension persists despite attempts to restore intravascular volume, ventricular preload must be further assessed. In patients with normal left ventricular function, the central venous pressure estimates ventricular preload. However, in the presence of left ventricular dysfunction, the central venous pressure is not an accurate guide to ventricular filling pressure, and a flow-directed pulmonary artery catheter should be inserted. During this time, administration of a vasopressor agent prevents a prolonged period of hypotension while hemodynamic monitoring is established. After insertion of the pulmonary artery catheter, left ventricular preload can be assessed by examining the pulmonary capillary wedge pressure (PCWP). The pulmonary artery catheter also allows for bedside measurement of cardiac output (CO) by the thermodilution technique. Hypovolemic shock is characterized by a low PCWP ($<$5 to 10 mm Hg) with a normal to low cardiac index (normal, 2.5 to 4.0 L•(min^{-1}•(m^{-2}) and a normal or elevated systemic vascular resistance (normal, 900 to 1,400 dyne•(s(•-cm^{-5}) defined as the following:

$$SVR = (MAP - CVP)/CO \times 80$$

where SVR is systemic vascular resistance, MAP is mean arterial pressure, CVP is central venous pressure, and CO is the measured cardiac output.

Cardiogenic shock is characterized by increased PCWP ($>$15 mm Hg) with a low cardiac index and elevated SVR. Patients in whom left ventricular failure is suspected should have an ECG and chemical analysis of the cardiac enzymes, including a fractionated creatinine phosphokinase (CPK) and troponin A, to rule out myocardial infarction. In septic shock PCWP is usually low with a very high CO and low SVR.

Treatment of such prolonged hypotension is now guided by following the variables of ventricular preload, CO, and urinary output. Hypovolemic shock is treated by intravenous administration of blood and crystalloid.

Cardiogenic shock is managed by first optimizing the ventricular preload. Although the heart normally functions with a low preload (PCWP, 3 to 8 mm Hg), when the left ventricle fails, it often functions best when the preload is elevated. Therefore, one should attempt to give fluid or blood intravenously to increase the preload and monitor the CO and stroke volume (SV):

$$CO = HR \times SV$$

where HR is heart rate.

Most patients have an optimal CO when the PCWP is increased to 15 to 20 mm Hg. Occasionally, patients with severe, long-standing ventricular failure require PCWP of 20 to 25 mm Hg to maintain CO. In addition to an optimal preload, these patients may also require inotropic support. Combined inotropic and vasopressor support often restores CO to near-normal values. Vasodilators should only be used in this setting if the hypotension has been first reversed with fluid and inotropic therapy.

Septic shock is managed by replacing the fluid lost from capillary endothelial leak with crystalloid. An inotropic agent such as dopamine is often added to increase CO further and to raise the arterial blood pressure. In unresponsive patients an α-adrenergic agonist, such as norepinephrine or phenylephrine, should be introduced.

HYPERTENSION

When hypertension develops in the PACU, it is often caused by pain, hypercapnia, hypoxemia, or excessive intravascular fluid volume. Any patient who manifests hypertension in the PACU should have these causes investigated and treated. Severe hypertension can lead to left ventricular failure, myocardial infarction, or a dysrhythmia from a sharp increase in myocardial oxygen consumption. Acute hypertension may also precipitate acute pulmonary edema or a cerebral hemorrhage. Preexisting hypertension is present in many patients who develop hypertension in the recovery room, and this is exacerbated if antihypertensive medications were abruptly withdrawn preoperatively.

Treatment of acute hypertension involves first treating the pain, hypercapnia, hypoxemia, or fluid overload. Persistent hypertension requires antihypertensive medication and as most postoperative hypertension usually resolves within 4 hours of surgery, long-acting antihypertensive drugs are unnecessary. A rapid-acting drug such as sodium nitroprusside is effective in treating postoperative hypertension because of its prompt onset and short duration of action. Nitroprusside is a vasodilator that acts directly on the vessel walls, both of the arterioles and venules, and is administered by continuous infusion beginning at 0.5 to 1.0 μg/kg per minute and titrated to an acceptable blood pressure. The dose should not exceed 10 μg/kg per minute or a total of 3 mg/kg in 24 hours, because the nitroprusside metabolite cyanide may cause toxicity from general blockade of oxidative phosphorylation, resulting in diffuse cellular hypoxic injury.

β-Blocking drugs such as propranolol, labetalol, and esmolol are also effective in treating hypertension during recovery. Labetalol, a combined α-blocking and β-blocking agent, is commonly used in the PACU. When used for treatment of postoperative hypertension, its β-blocking effects predominate, and the reduction in blood pressure results from its negative inotropic effects. Labetalol can be given in intravenous 5-mg increments, with the effect on blood pressure apparent in several minutes. Esmolol is an ultrashort-acting β-blocker that may be given as a continuous infusion at rates of 25 to 300 µg/kg per minute .

DYSRHYTHMIAS

The factors predisposing to development of postoperative dysrhythmias include electrolyte imbalance (especially hypokalemia), hypoxia, hypercapnia, metabolic alkalosis and acidosis, and preexisting heart disease. When a dysrhythmia occurs in the PACU, it is often a sign of a metabolic or a perfusion-related problem. Dysrhythmias appearing in the PACU rarely need long-term treatment. The most common dysrhythmias are sinus tachycardia, sinus bradycardia, ventricular premature beats, ventricular tachycardia, and supraventricular tachyarrhythmias.

MYOCARDIAL ISCHEMIA

The postoperative patient who complains of chest pain suggestive of acute myocardial ischemia must undergo a prompt and targeted evaluation. Classic symptoms include substernal chest pain with radiation to the shoulders, neck, arms, or back, and lightheadedness, sweating, nausea, and dyspnea, often accompanied by a feeling of distress, anxiety, or impending doom. One should immediately assess vital signs (including oxygen saturation), obtain intravenous access, and perform a 12-lead ECG. After review of the patient's history, serum cardiac marker levels, electrolyte, and coagulation studies should be performed and a portable chest x-ray obtained.

Immediate general treatment includes oxygen, aspirin 325 mg (unless surgically contraindicated), and nitroglycerin sublingual or by inhaled spray. Morphine may be given for chest pain not relieved by nitroglycerin.

Evaluation of the 12-lead ECG focuses on looking for either (1) ST-segment elevation or new left bundle branch block, or (2) ST-segment depression or T-wave inversion.

Patients with ST-segment elevation require urgent attention as they are at significant risk for myocardial infarction and cardiac failure. These patients usually undergo rapid reperfusion therapy, either using fibrinolytic drugs or by performing coronary angioplasty and stent placement. Adjunctive therapy often includes β-blockers and angiotensin-converting enzyme inhibitors. Recent surgery represents a potential contraindication to the use of intravenous fibrinolytic agents, and in these patients coronary angioplasty with stent placement is usually the better option. If signs of cardiogenic shock are present, immediate percutaneous coronary intervention with angioplasty or stent placement is indicated.

Patients with ST-segment depression are usually treated with intravenous nitroglycerin and heparin, aspirin, β-blockers, and glycoprotein IIb/IIIa inhibitors.

Failure To Regain Consciousness

The patient who does not regain consciousness after general anesthesia requires a careful evaluation. Preoperative factors such as drug or alcohol intoxication should be sought. The most common reason for persistent somnolence is residual effects of anesthetics, sedatives, and preoperative medications. In most such cases, some level of responsiveness should occur within 90 minutes after emergence from the anesthesia. Initial management should include pharmacologic reversal agents aimed at the most likely sedative drug. Naloxone in small doses (0.2 mg intravenous) will increase ventilatory rate if narcotic sedation is the problem. Physostigmine (1.25 mg intravenous) can reverse the effects of some sedatives and inhalation anesthetics. The sedative and amnestic effects of the benzodiazepines can be reversed by the use of flumazenil (up to 1.0 mg intravenous). Profound neuromuscular blockade can mimic unconsciousness, and this must also be excluded.

Second, once pharmacologic causes are ruled out, metabolic reasons must be sought. Profound hypothermia (temperature $< 33°C$) can produce unconsciousness, as can profound hypoglycemia or hyperglycemia. Blood glucose, electrolytes, and blood gases should be evaluated in all such cases. If there is reason to suspect hypoglycemia, 50% dextrose should be administered intravenously before a blood glucose determination.

Third, if the diagnosis remains unclear, a structural neurologic abnormality should be sought. Raised intracranial pressure may occur after head trauma or neurosurgery. Thromboembolic and hemorrhagic cerebrovascular accidents can occur in the postoperative period, but they are uncommon. Intraoperative cerebral hypoxia from hypoxemia or poor cerebral perfusion can produce a diffuse encephalopathy. Emergency computed tomography scanning is used to evaluate the presence of raised intracranial pressure or an acute intracranial cause of the delayed emergence.

Rarely, a local anesthetic overdose can present as unconsciousness. Old age per se does not usually account for delayed emergence from general anesthesia.

Pain and Agitation

Postoperative pain and agitation are common problems (see Chapter 17). Pain can usually be controlled using small doses of intravenous opioids; however, certain patients need large doses of narcotics to control severe pain. In addition, patients occasionally awaken from anesthesia in a violent, agitated state. Although this type of exaggerated response may be caused by pain, several other important factors could be involved. Hypoxemia, hypercapnia, gastric distension, and urinary retention with bladder distension can all result in marked agitation. The use of scopolamine, phenothiazines, and barbiturates as premedicants without narcotics increases the incidence of postoperative excitement.

Management of the agitated patient involves ascertaining the adequacy of the vital signs and blood gas exchange, excluding urinary or gastric distension, and administering a small dose of intravenous narcotic.

Many factors influence the onset, incidence, and severity of postoperative pain. The age of the patient is important, with the very young and very old seeming to experience less pain than do those in the middle years of life. The site of the operation influences the severity of pain, with thoracotomy being, in general, the most painful operation, and upper abdominal surgery a close second. Lower abdominal surgery is usually less painful.

Most cases of postoperative pain can be managed by giving small intravenous doses of narcotics. Narcotics for pain relief result in a decreased tidal volume, and a slow regular pattern of respiration. The presence of pain does not prevent narcotic-induced respiratory depression, so these patients need encouragement to cough and to breathe deeply. Patients in pain can be given 2 to 5 mg of morphine every 15 to 30 minutes with careful observation of the degree of pain relief and the amount of respiratory depression.

Continuous infusion of narcotic analgesics results in a smoother course when these agents are used for postoperative pain relief, and although patients maintain constant blood levels of analgesic and receive less total drug dose, these infusions require careful monitoring and titration. Patient-controlled analgesia (PCA), the self-administration of small doses of opioids by patients when they experience pain, is designed to minimize the effects of pharmacokinetic and pharmacodynamic variability among individual patients. When the patient triggers the PCA pump, a preset incremental dose of opioid is delivered into the patient's intravenous catheter. The PCA technique allows the patient to determine the timing of analgesic doses and allows for improved titration of analgesia, and also minimizes patient anxiety.

The use of narcotics in the epidural space to control postoperative pain is also a very effective approach. Epidural morphine (2 to 4 mg diluted to 10 mL) provides prompt analgesia with a duration of approximately 12 hours. Complications include respiratory depression, which is dose related and can occur as long as 6 hours after injection. Significant respiratory depression occurs in less than 1% of patients receiving epidural narcotics and is reversible with naloxone. Fentanyl and sufentanil have also been used successfully for epidural analgesia, but approximately 15% to 20% of patients complain of pruritus. Nausea and urinary retention have also been reported. These techniques are most useful for patients having major thoracic or abdominal surgery and at high risk for complications of parenteral analgesic therapy.

Continuous epidural block using mixtures of short-acting narcotics and dilute local anesthetic solutions can provide excellent postoperative analgesia and, when administered in the thoracic space, can permit early postoperative ambulation.

Nonnarcotic analgesics are being used increasingly for postoperative pain. The most common agents used are the nonsteroidal anti-inflammatory agents. Ketorolac was among the first to be available for parenteral administration and is free of respiratory depressant effects. Although ketorolac is not as potent as the narcotics, it can be an effective adjunct or alternative to narcotic analgesics without major complications. Anecdotal concerns about ketorolac center on the possibility of increased bleeding in patients receiving this agent; however, well-controlled evaluations of this potential problem are lacking at this time. Finally, ibuprofen has been suggested as a reasonable alternative to narcotic analgesics in patients undergoing laparoscopic surgery. Newer, more-specific nonsteroidal intravenous agents are being studied, and may become available in the near future.

Postoperative Nausea and Vomiting

Postoperative nausea and vomiting (PONV) are common complications that result in patient discomfort, prolonged stay in the PACU, and, rarely, pulmonary aspiration or incisional disruption. They are often multifactorial in origin, and there is little strong evidence that any one anesthetic technique has a lower incidence of nausea and vomiting than others, except that the sedative and hypnotic propofol appears to have an inherent antiemetic effect. Opiates are associated with nausea and vomiting, especially when used as the predominant part of the anesthetic. The type of surgical procedure also has an important influence on the occurrence of nausea and vomiting, with patients having laparoscopic, middle ear, and strabismus surgery at increased risk for this complication.

Hypothermia

Inadvertent hypothermia is a common occurrence after major surgical procedures. The major adverse effects are patient discomfort, vasoconstriction, and shivering. Full recovery may take many hours. Shivering increases metabolic rate and hence the need to increase CO and minute ventilation. Longer anesthetics are associated with a higher frequency of shivering. Prevention is important, and the use of a heated humidifier and forced-air heated blankets results in a higher patient temperature on arrival in the PACU. Once in the PACU, hypothermic patients should receive supplemental oxygen, warmed intravenous fluids and blood, and external warming devices. Although many drugs have been used to treat postanesthetic shivering, meperidine (12.5 to 25 mg intravenous) is effective in both stopping the shivering and decreasing oxygen consumption.

SUMMARY

The degree of physiologic stress related to surgical procedures has a direct impact on the recovery and rehabilitation of our patients, and this principle is often acutely demonstrated in the PACU. Therefore, care provided in the PACU is of key importance to patients as the early diagnosis and management of postoperative complications may exert a significant influence on overall surgical outcome. Also, with the continuing rise in the ambulatory surgery population, the optimal management of patients in the PACU will increasingly influence the overall perioperative and hospital experience.

SUGGESTED READINGS

Rose DK, Cohen MM, DeBoer DP. Cardiovascular events in the postanesthesia care unit: contribution of risk factors. Anesthesiology 1996; 772-781.

Ganong WF. Respiratory Adjustments in Health and Disease, In Ganong WF, ed. Review of medical physiology Columbus: McGraw-Hill, 2001; 658-673.

Lumb AB. Anaesthesia. In: Lumb AB, ed. Nunn's Applied Respiratory Physiology. Oxford: Butterworth-Heinemann Medical, 1999; 420-452.

Mecca RS, Postoperative recovery. in Barash PG, et al ed. Clinical Anesthesia. Philadelphia: Lippincott Williams and Wilkins, 1997; 1279-1304.

CHAPTER 13

Putting It All Together:
An Anesthesia Case Study

Randall S. Glidden, MD

The preceding chapters introduced the basics of anesthesiology. Although it is convenient to divide our knowledge base into various topics, such division is somewhat arbitrary and artificial. In reality the daily practice of anesthesiology requires us to draw on this knowledge base as a whole and extract all that is necessary to best serve the particular needs of each patient that we care for.

To best illustrate this, we will turn our attention to the anesthetic management of a much more complicated patient than Mr. Morton whom we met in Chapter 2. Although this patient will proceed through the same "steps" from preoperative assessment to recovery from anesthesia, you will note a marked qualitative difference in complexity from Mr. Morton's "simple anesthetic."

THE PATIENT AND HIS OPERATION

Mr. Wells is a 57-year-old man with localized, asymptomatic colon cancer found on routine colonoscopy who is scheduled for a right colectomy in 2 weeks.

STEP 1: THE PREOPERATIVE EVALUATION

As we discussed in Chapter 2, the preoperative evaluation begins with a history and physical examination.

You learn that Mr. Wells' medical history includes the following significant problems:

1. *Insulin-dependent diabetes mellitus (IDDM) × 23 years.*
2. *Coronary artery disease (CAD), status post myocardial infarction in 1996, and status post coronary artery bypass grafting (CABG) × 4 in 1996. He gets occasional angina with exertion.*
3. *Hypertension.*
4. *Chronic obstructive pulmonary disease (COPD), probably secondary to smoking two packs of cigarettes a day for 42 years.*
5. *Hiatal hernia with reflux.*
6. *Chronic renal insufficiency secondary to diabetes; a recent creatinine was 1.9 mg/dL.*

His surgical history includes CABG in 1996 and appendectomy in 1965, both under general anesthesia. He denies any problems with his anesthetics.

He has no allergies, and his medications include insulin, atenolol, lisinopril, diltiazem, omeprazole, and an albuterol metered-dose inhaler.

On physical examination you find the following:

Height 5′8″, weight 200 pounds, blood pressure 184/93 mm Hg, pulse 87 beats/min, and respiratory rate 20 breaths/min.

He is moderately obese, and appears to be in no acute distress.

When he opens his mouth and sticks out his tongue you can see only his hard palate, but his teeth are intact. His neck extension is normal, and his mentum to hyoid distance is two fingers' breadths. His lungs sound clear, and he has normal heart sounds without murmurs.

Questions:

1. What are Mr. Wells's most significant problems for the anesthesiologist?
2. What laboratory tests would you order at this time?
3. Does Mr. Wells need anything else before he goes to surgery?
4. Which medications should he take on the morning of his surgery?

You believe that Mr. Wells's most significant problems include active CAD and hypertension, IDDM, COPD, reflux, and possibly a difficult airway. Because his CAD is active he is at risk for perioperative myocardial ischemia or infarction. Also, diabetes may mask anginal symptoms making perioperative diagnosis difficult. His pulmonary disease poses a risk of bronchospasm, ventilation–perfusion imbalance, and perioperative problems with oxygenation and ventilation. He has a Mallampati class III airway and active reflux, which increases the risk of both difficulty with intubation and aspiration of stomach contents.

You order a complete blood count (CBC), electrolyte panel with glucose, blood urea nitrogen (BUN), and creatinine; 12-lead electrocardiogram (ECG); and a posteroanterior chest radiograph.

Because Mr. Wells has had no recent evaluation of his cardiac status, you refer him to a cardiologist for further evaluation. The cardiologist will probably order additional studies to assess cardiac function and risk for myocardial ischemia or infarction.

You tell Mr. Wells to take all of his usual medications on the morning of surgery; however, you tell him to reduce by half his usual morning insulin dose.

You obtain Mr. Wells's informed consent for anesthesia for his operation, but you tell him that final plans for anesthetic management will depend on the results of his laboratory tests and cardiology consultation and will be discussed on the morning of his surgery.

On the day before his operation you review Mr. Wells's laboratory studies and the note from the cardiologist. His CBC showed normal hemoglobin and hematocrit values (14 gm/dL and 42%, respectively), his glucose was 193 mg/dL, his BUN was 16 mg/dL, and his creatinine was 1.8 mg/dL. His ECG showed sinus rhythm with a rate of 73, anterior and inferior Q waves (consistent with an old anterior-inferior myocardial infarction), but no ST-segment depression. His chest radiograph revealed a slightly enlarged heart and mildly hyperinflated lungs, consistent with COPD.

The cardiologist had ordered an echocardiogram, which showed fair left ventricular function and an ejection fraction of 47%. He also ordered a thallium-stress test, which was positive for ST-segment depression in the lateral chest leads without angina during exercise; thallium images showed lateral reperfusion after exercise, indicative of an area of myocardium at risk for ischemia. He recommended continuing all of Mr. Wells's medications and that he have "close monitoring of blood pressure and ECG" during the surgery.

Questions

Based on a now complete preoperative data base:

1. What major perioperative problems do you anticipate?
2. Should Mr. Wells have general or spinal anesthesia?
3. What intraoperative monitors will you use?
4. How will you manage his postoperative pain?

Mr. Wells's further workup confirmed your previous concerns about the risk of perioperative ischemia, so you will plan your anesthetic in a way that maximizes myocardial oxygen delivery and minimizes myocardial oxygen demand. You still have concerns about Mr. Wells's airway and aspiration potential, and his diabetes, mild COPD, and renal insufficiency add to his overall risk. You don't anticipate large blood losses, but this operation could produce considerable "third-space" losses.

Although one could use spinal anesthesia for a right colectomy, you decide that general anesthesia will probably give you more control of hemodynamics and ventilation. In addition to the routine monitors used during all anesthetics, you decide to place a radial artery catheter so you can follow his blood pressure more closely and treat hypertension or hypotension more quickly than you could using a blood pressure cuff alone.

Because pain can lead to postoperative myocardial ischemia and infarction, you plan to place a thoracic epidural catheter before induction. You will infuse a low-dose mixture of bupivacaine and fentanyl through the catheter during Mr. Wells's surgery and then continue the infusion through the first few postoperative days.

You fall asleep that night thinking about all the details of Mr. Wells's operation in the morning.

STEP 2: PATIENT PREPARATION I
(PREOPERATIVE HOLDING AREA)

The next day Mr. Wells arrives at 6:30 for his 8:00 operation. The nurse in the preoperative holding area confirms his nil per os (NPO) status, asks about morning medications, checks his vital signs, and has him put on a hospital gown. She learns that he took all his medications and took half his insulin as instructed. His vital signs are similar to those from his preoperative visit, including a heart rate of 83 beats/min and a blood pressure of 178/89 mm Hg.

Mr. Wells appears nervous, but he remembers you from the preoperative clinic and is happy to see you. You go over your concerns with him about his cardiac and other risk factors. He agrees with your plan to put in an intravenous (IV) catheter and an arterial line, and to place a thoracic epidural (for intraoperative analgesia as well as for postoperative pain control) before going into the operating room. General anesthesia is just fine with him because he wants "to be out" for the surgery.

You insert a 16-gauge catheter in a left forearm vein (large anticipated fluid requirement) and then give him 2 mg of midazolam and 50 mg of fentanyl. Next you cannulate the left radial artery and place the thoracic epidural catheter without any difficulty.

Before you take him into the operating room you confirm that Mr. Wells has a current sample of blood in the blood bank and that a "type and screen" has been performed.

STEP 3: PATIENT PREPARATION II (OPERATING ROOM)

At 7:43 the surgeon, Dr. Cushing, arrives. After she answers a few of his last-minute questions, you wheel Mr. Wells into the operating room. He moves onto the operating room table, and you attach the ECG leads, pulse oximeter, a noninvasive blood pressure cuff, and a peripheral nerve stimulator. You attach the arterial catheter to the line connected to the arterial pressure transducer. You confirm that you see a good arterial pressure waveform, all the monitors are working properly, and the IV line is running well. You attach the IV line to a fluid warmer.

As you prepare to preoxygenate Mr. Wells you inspect the anesthesia machine one more time. If you have trouble with the intubation you have an emergency airway cart with a fiberoptic bronchoscope set up and ready to go.

STEP 4: INDUCTION OF ANESTHESIA I

Questions:

1. In light of Mr. Wells's cardiac history, how will you induce anesthesia without producing potentially detrimental perturbations of hemodynamics?

2. *Given Mr. Wells's possible difficult airway, how will you induce*
   anesthesia in such a way that minimizes the risk of hypoxemia,
   aspiration, or failed intubation?

   You ask Mr. Wells to breathe deeply through the oxygen mask you
   placed on his face. This preoxygenation will reduce the risk of hypox-
   emia during induction, especially if intubation proves difficult or pro-
   longed. You slowly inject 250 mg of fentanyl IV, which should blunt
   the hemodynamic response to intubation, and you also inject 50 mg
   of esmolol (a short-acting β-blocker) to help prevent an increase in
   heart rate. You attach a syringe of sodium pentothal to the IV line. Pen-
   tothal will induce rapid loss of consciousness, and because of its
   myocardial depressant effects, it will further help blunt hypertension
   during induction.

   Because of Mr. Wells's history of hiatal hernia and reflux, you per-
   form a "rapid sequence induction." As you inject the pentothal, an
   assistant presses down on the cricoid cartilage, thus compressing the
   esophagus and preventing passive gastroesophageal reflux. Immedi-
   ately after the pentothal injection you inject 100 mg of succinyl-
   choline to produce rapid paralysis. Unlike a standard induction, you
   do not attempt to ventilate the lungs before paralysis, as this could
   induce regurgitation. Cricoid pressure will be maintained until you
   have confirmed that the endotracheal tube is in the trachea.

STEP 5: AIRWAY MANAGEMENT

You attempt laryngoscopy with a Macintosh 3 blade, but all you can
see is the tip of the epiglottis. You try various maneuvers to bring the
vocal cords into view without success. The arterial oxygen saturation
(SaO$_2$) is 96% and falling.

Question:

1. *What do you do now?*

   As you reach for an oral airway you ask the nurse to call another
   anesthesiologist into the room. With the oxygen saturation falling you
   must establish ventilation as soon as possible. You insert the oral air-
   way and, much to your relief, you find that you can ventilate the
   lungs. Your assistant continues to hold cricoid pressure as Dr. Bier, the
   anesthesia "floor leader," comes into the room. After you give sever-
   al positive-pressure breaths, Dr. Bier assists you as you quickly pass
   the fiberoptic bronchoscope into Mr. Wells's trachea. You slide an
   endotracheal tube over the bronchoscope and into the trachea and
   then remove the bronchoscope, leaving the tube in place. A few
   breaths confirm proper placement, and you tape the tube in place.
   The SaO$_2$, which had fallen to 83%, rises to 100% after restoring ven-
   tilation. You glance at the arterial tracing and are relieved to see that
   despite the potential stress of this difficult intubation, Mr. Wells's

blood pressure is 166/82 mm Hg and his heart rate is 72 beats/min. You take a few deep breaths yourself as relative calm returns to the operating room.

STEP 6: INDUCTION OF ANESTHESIA II

With intubation complete you turn on nitrous oxide and isoflurane to continue the anesthetic induction. You plan on using the infusion of low-dose bupivacaine and fentanyl through the epidural catheter as a means of producing intraoperative analgesia, but in addition the inhaled agents will maintain hypnosis and amnesia and should further blunt hemodynamic responses to surgical stimulation. You attach the epidural catheter to a syringe pump and start infusing the local anesthetic and narcotic mixture.

After the peripheral nerve stimulator shows the return of twitches (thus confirming metabolism of succinylcholine), you slowly inject 6 mg of vecuronium IV. Because pancuronium can cause an increase in heart rate and its effect is prolonged in patients with renal insufficiency, you feel that vecuronium is a better choice for Mr. Wells.

STEP 7: MAINTENANCE OF ANESTHESIA

With induction complete, the operating room circulating nurse inserts a urinary catheter into Mr. Wells's bladder. Dr. Cushing preps and drapes the operative field. You place an upper extremity warm-air blanket and insert a nasopharyngeal temperature probe. The anesthesia agent analyzer shows that the nitrous oxide–isoflurane mixture is at 1 MAC (minimal alveolar concentration).

Dr. Cushing makes her incision and begins Mr. Wells's colectomy. Mr. Wells's pulse is 62 beats/min and his blood pressure is 136/71 mm Hg.

All goes well for approximately an hour when you notice that quite a large amount of blood is suddenly flowing into the suction canister. Dr. Cushing tells you that "there's a little bleeding here." The blood pressure is now 97/63 mm Hg, the heart rate is 114 beats/min, the SaO_2 is 97%, and you notice a 2-mm ST-segment depression in lead V_5.

Questions:

1. How much IV fluid should you have given by this point in the operation?
2. How much IV fluid should you give now to replace the blood loss?
3. When should you transfuse with blood?
4. What do you do about the ECG changes?

At the start of the operation you calculated Mr. Wells's fluid deficit to be approximately 1 L because he had been NPO for 8 hours (see Chapter 9). You calculated third-space loss to be roughly 6 mL/kg per hour or approximately 600 mL. You had replaced the calculated deficit and losses with 1500 mL of lactated Ringer's solution before the sudden blood loss, and urine output had been adequate at 60 mL during the hour.

You see that the suction canister contains blood up to the 600-mL mark, so you are now infusing lactated Ringer's solution as fast as you can using a pressurized sleeve over the IV fluid bag. You calculate that you will need to infuse approximately 2 L of isotonic IV fluid to make up for the acute blood loss (3:1, crystalloid to blood). Because Mr. Wells's starting hematocrit was 42%, you feel that you probably won't need to transfuse packed red blood cells unless he loses approximately 2000 mL of blood (calculated allowable blood loss to reach a Hct of 30%).

The ST-segment depression may be caused by a combination of mild hypotension and tachycardia, leading to a decrease in myocardial oxygen delivery relative to increased oxygen demand. After increasing the fraction of inspired oxygen (F_{IO_2}) to 100%, you try to restore intravascular volume to normal with IV fluid, and you give 50 mg of phenylephrine to increase the blood pressure. In addition you start an infusion of nitroglycerin to provide coronary vasodilation, realizing that more phenylephrine may need to be given to counter a potential nitroglycerin-induced drop in blood pressure. You also consider giving esmolol if necessary to slow the heart rate, but increasing intravascular volume is your first goal. You send a blood specimen for stat hematocrit and glucose, because tachycardia can be related to anemia or hypoglycemia.

The combination of IV fluid (total given, 3500 mL) and phenylephrine bring the blood pressure up to 136/72 mm Hg and the heart rate decreases to 102 beats/min. The laboratory calls to tell you that his hematocrit is 36%, but his glucose is only 48 mg/dL. You give 50 mL of 50% dextrose solution. The heart rate slows to 77 beats/min, and the ST segments revert to normal as Dr. Cushing announces that she has controlled the bleeding and is beginning to close the abdomen.

STEP 8: EMERGENCE FROM ANESTHESIA

You lower the inspired concentration of isoflurane as Dr. Cushing closes. Once the fascial layer is closed, you reverse the vecuronium neuromuscular blockade with neostigmine and glycopyrrolate. You decrease the minute ventilation and allow the end-tidal CO_2 to rise so that Mr. Wells will begin to breathe spontaneously. As Dr. Cushing closes the skin, Mr. Wells is breathing with a 300-mL tidal volume and a rate of 16 breaths/min. His blood pressure and heart rate are 136/78 mm Hg and 63 beats/min, respectively, as you turn off the nitrous oxide and isoflurane. Soon Mr. Wells opens his eyes, and you suction his oropharynx and remove his endotracheal tube. He is sleepy but responsive and denies having any pain. You move him to the stretcher, give him oxygen to breathe by face mask, and continue to monitor his arterial blood pressure as you transport him to the postanesthesia care unit (PACU).

STEP 9: RECOVERY FROM ANESTHESIA

In the PACU Mr. Wells's vital signs are in their normal range. He is drowsy but responsive, and he has no pain. You continue the infusion through his epidural catheter. Although his ECG tracing on the PACU monitor looks normal, you order a 12-lead ECG and cardiac enzyme studies to follow up the ischemic episode in the operating room and to rule out myocardial infarction.

As the recovery room nurse is attaching the leads for the ECG you ordered, Mr. Wells suddenly looks rather pale and is somnolent. You are called stat to the PACU where you find his blood pressure is 77/44 mm Hg, his heart rate is 126 beats/min, and he has a 4-mm ST-segment elevation on the ECG monitor and frequent multifocal premature ventricular contractions. The 12-lead ECG confirms these acute changes.

Questions:

1. What do you think is going on?
2. What do you do first?
3. What further action should you take?

You correctly deduce that Mr. Wells is having a myocardial ischemic event (now referred to as an acute coronary syndrome), probably with rapidly developing cardiogenic shock. This could be secondary to an acute thrombosis of a coronary artery, so it demands your immediate attention. Because of his diabetes and his thoracic epidural, he may have ischemia without chest pain.

First you optimize oxygenation with mask oxygen, noting that the SaO$_2$ rises from 94% to 99%. You ask for a stat cardiology consultation, and you begin an infusion of phenylephrine to raise the blood pressure and improve myocardial perfusion pressure and nitroglycerin to maximize coronary vasodilation. As the blood pressure improves, you give IV metoprolol to slow the heart rate and 325 mg of aspirin by rectal suppository.

The combination of phenylephrine, nitroglycerin, and metoprolol raises Mr. Wells's blood pressure to 110/68 mm Hg and slows his heart rate to 73 beats/min, and his mental status improves. He now admits to some chest pressure so you give him small doses of morphine IV as the cardiologist arrives.

Within 20 minutes Mr. Wells is in the cardiac catheterization suite undergoing angioplasty and stent placement for an occluded left anterior descending coronary artery.

After the procedure Mr Wells's cardiac enzyme studies show that he had a myocardial infarction. However, his ECG reverts to baseline status, indicative of a (probably less severe) subendocardial myocardial infarction. Mr. Wells has an otherwise uneventful recovery from his colectomy and coronary stent placement. He is discharged from the hospital on the tenth postoperative day.

SUMMARY

During the day-to-day practice of our specialty, the anesthesiologist must often draw on a vast knowledge base to give optimal care to patients suffering from a variety of medical conditions during a multitude of different surgical procedures. Sometimes our anesthetic plan must be altered to meet individual patient needs, which may include an escalation of care necessitated by the not infrequent occurrence of life-threatening illness or complications. Whether relatively simple or exceedingly complex, anesthetic management proceeds through orderly steps in which diligence of practice and attention to details usually precede satisfactory outcomes.

SUGGESTED READING

Cummins RO, ed. Advanced Cardiac Life Support (ACLS) Provider Manual. Dallas: American Heart Association, 2001.

PART II

ANESTHESIOLOGY SPECIALTY AREAS

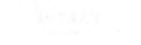

CHAPTER 14

Ambulatory Anesthesia

Lisa L. Lombard, MD

GENERAL INFORMATION AND HISTORY

In this era of managed health care there is a steadily increasing trend to perform outpatient procedures driven by the need to lower health-care costs and increase operating room efficiency. Ambulatory anesthesia has its roots, however, not from the current financial health-care crisis, but instead from the early twentieth-century desire to increase patient satisfaction. By 1909, James Nicoll, MD, had already performed nearly 9000 outpatient pediatric procedures at the Glasgow Royal Hospital for sick children. The first American freestanding surgicenter for minor surgical and dental cases, the Downtown Anesthesia Clinic, was opened in 1916 by Ralph Waters, MD, in Sioux City, Iowa. His prediction that many surgeons would be opening post-World War I minor surgical clinics attests to his foresight that patients would eventually prefer small procedures performed away from the larger and more-threatening hospitals. Although the Society for the Advancement of Freestanding Ambulatory Surgical Centers was established in 1974, it was a decade later that the Society for Ambulatory Anesthesia (SAMBA) was organized. Twenty anesthesiologists met during the 1984 American Society of Anesthesiologists meeting and formed this fledgling society dedicated to the education and research needs of perioperative physicians practicing ambulatory anesthesia.

SELECTION CRITERIA

How do we select which patients are good candidates for ambulatory surgery? This is best seen in two perspectives: patient criteria and procedure criteria.

Patient Criteria

The overall medical condition of the patient is probably the most important concern. As you learned in Chapter 8, all patients are divided into an ASA physical status classification I through V. Usually ASA class I or II patients are preferred for outpatient procedures; however, ASA class III or IV patients may be acceptable if their medical condition is stable or optimally managed. Patient age seems a natural selection criterion; however, it is useful only in the pediatric population. There are no advanced age restrictions and in fact many nonagenarians undergo cataract surgery and occasionally we see some centenarians. Evaluation of elderly patients instead focuses on the physiologic age in terms of medical illnesses and ASA classification.

In formerly premature infants, the evaluation must assess the postconceptual age (PCA) and the infant's risk of apnea. If there have been recent apneic spells or the PCA is younger than 50 weeks, one might prefer to perform the surgery in a center that can admit the child for overnight observation after the procedure.

All patients must have a reliable escort to accompany them home and to help them settle in after their surgery. It is preferred that they also have help through the night; however, depending on surgical procedure, it may be acceptable to at least have someone nearby that they can call for help, such as a neighbor.

A preoperative screening determines final suitability for outpatient surgery. Whether this is done by a telephone interview, a visit to the preoperative clinic, or online, a nurse or physician must review the patient's medical and surgical history, medication use, proposed procedure, and escort status at least 24 hours before the procedure. This also allows the staff to confirm nil per os (NPO) status and arrival time, and to address any special-care needs the patient may have.

Procedure Criteria

Although we seem to keep pushing the envelope in terms of the complexity of procedures performed on an outpatient basis, the type of facility in which the surgery is performed is still the most important factor. Not all surgeries are performed in a hospital or surgicenter setting; some may be performed in the surgeon's office. Office-based procedures often are the least invasive with anesthesia usually consisting of local anesthetics with or without conscious sedation or monitored anesthesia care. These are frequently minor plastic or dermatologic procedures that do not invade any body cavity. Emergency medical backup in this type of facility is usually provided by local 911 service or ambulance to the nearest hospital.

Surgical suites may also exist in clinics designed especially for ambulatory procedures and occasionally procedures requiring an overnight observation. These freestanding clinics or surgicenters must have equipment and personnel to provide advanced cardiac life support (ACLS) if necessary, but should only commence procedures that have a low risk for significant blood loss or surgical complication that might need a larger corrective surgery. These facilities frequently have no or very limited blood banks and usually do not have additional experienced surgeons that can assist in case of an emergency. It is best not to perform intrathoracic procedures such as thoracoscopy or thoracic biopsies in such a facility unless exquisitely set up to handle major complications; these are perhaps best performed in a surgicenter attached to a hospital so that the patient with a significant complication has access to a plethora of additional personnel and equipment.

In general, the procedures for ambulatory patients should:

1. Be of relatively short duration so that the patient has adequate time for recovery and travel home.
2. Produce minimal physiologic alteration.
3. Have a low risk of significant blood loss.
4. Be of limited invasiveness to body cavities (usually one organ).
5. Not consist of multiple procedures.
6. Require minimal postoperative care and produce minimal postoperative discomfort.
7. Present a low risk for hidden postoperative complications (such as airway swelling or perforated viscus).

PREOPERATIVE PREPARATION AND PREMEDICATION

As with any anesthetic, the goal is a plan that takes into account optimum patient safety and insensibility to pain according to the patient's needs and preexisting medical problems, one that will optimize surgical conditions, and provide a smooth emergence and uneventful recovery. The goals of the patient, surgeon, and anesthesiologist must be the same. For example, the best-performed ambulatory anesthetic will fail if the patient's goal is to stay overnight in the hospital. Instead, we strive to restore postsurgical patients to nearly the same condition we observed on their arrival.

With this in mind, the most important step is the bedside history and physical examination followed by a discussion of these goals with the patient. The only thing that makes ambulatory anesthesia unique is that the patient returns home on the same day, sometimes within just a few hours. If the practitioner keeps in mind the most common side effects of each procedure and makes a plan to minimize their impact on the patient, this will nearly always be successful.

After the NPO status and escort availability are confirmed, the history, physical, and consents obtained, and the intravenous line is inserted, it is time to consider premedication. This can take many forms. Some patients need only verbal anxiolysis and an escort to the operating room, others want "to be knocked out" at this time. For the latter patient reassurance of quality care and patient comfort measures together with a modest dose of an anxiolytic (e.g., midazolam) or a small dose of a hypnotic (e.g., propofol) is usually all that is necessary. In the ambulatory suite "less is better," as intravenous drugs such as benzodiazepines and narcotics may delay emergence from anesthesia and increase postanesthesia care unit (PACU) recovery time.

This is also a good time to give antibiotics necessary for the procedure, GI propulsive drugs (e.g., metoclopramide), nonparticulate antacids, or acid blockers. Peripheral nerve blocks for surgeries of the extremities can be performed at this time in the preoperative areas or preinduction rooms because they have monitors for blood pressure, pulse oximetry (SpO_2), and electrocardiogram, as well as the availability of oxygen delivery.

Preoperative narcotics can be given but with sufficient care and caution. When narcotic analgesia will be the main control of postoperative pain, many anesthesiologists prefer to titrate the narcotic as a premedication so that they can assess the potency in the patient. This is done with oxygen administration, SpO_2 monitoring, and constant bedside vigilance. If large doses of narcotics will be necessary for an outpatient surgery (such as anterior cruciate ligament repairs with autografts, or Bankhardt procedures in which regional anesthesia is contraindicated or refused), there is a benefit to front-loading the narcotic so as to minimize respiratory depression and sedation postoperatively.

ANESTHETIC MANAGEMENT

How do you decide what kind of anesthetic to give? General, regional, sedation, or local? Although many operations can only be performed under general anesthesia (e.g., tonsillectomy or cholecystectomy), others will allow you to choose the one best suited to the patient and surgeon. Much of this discussion overlaps with the art of medicine. Most anesthesiologists have a preference or style that suits them and can be altered when necessary. Many patients today come to the hospital requesting one technique that was suggested to them by their surgeons or Internet chat rooms. The art is in pleasing everybody while at the same time providing a safe and effective anesthetic.

Most surgeries of the limbs such as knee arthroscopy, bunion resection, or carpal tunnel release can be performed with regional anesthesia. Surgeries that invade the abdomen or thorax usually require general anesthesia. Pelvic surgeries can be performed using general, regional, or local anesthesia with conscious sedation. Superficial procedures like biopsies or cataracts can be done with local anesthesia with or without sedation. Besides patient and surgeon factors, cost and time for anesthetic recovery and operating room turnover also influence the choice of anesthetic.

Spinal anesthesia is making a resurgence in ambulatory centers. With the prior concerns of prolonged motor blockade, delayed voiding, postdural puncture headaches, and prolonged procedure starting times, anesthesiologists who favored regional anesthesia were often given a barrage of complaints. By lowering the dose of local anesthetic while adding small amounts of short-acting narcotics, anesthesiologists have been able to fine-tune the technique to minimize the aforementioned side effects. Postdural puncture headaches and delayed starting times can be minimized by using highly experienced staff.

Monitored anesthesia care (MAC) is a term now reserved for anesthetic management supplied by an anesthesiologist or certified nurse anesthetist (CRNA) (see also Chapter 7). This is a result of the arrival of operating room nurses who are trained to give small doses of medications called conscious sedation. Although monitored anesthesia care implies the use of sedatives, some patients are too ill to tolerate the side effects that sedatives can cause (e.g., cardiac or respiratory depression). For these patients it is necessary to have anesthesia personnel present to manage the potential medical derangements that the surgery may cause. This is monitored anesthesia care in its truest sense. When sedation medications *are* used, they provide short-term sedation or hypnosis and their effects need to cease when the procedure is finished. Short-acting agents such as midazolam, propofol, methohexital, fentanyl, and remifentanil are preferred because of their short duration and ease of titration.

General anesthesia, when chosen, needs to have a fast onset and fast offset. Anesthetic turnover, the time from when the last patient leaves the room until the next one enters, is usually 8 to 12 minutes in most surgicenters. It is difficult for a center to be profitable if this turnover time is too long. Thus agents have been developed with this pharmacologic profile in mind. A rapid and smooth induction is generally achieved with intravenous agents such as propofol or methohexital or by inhalation of sevoflurane in oxygen and nitrous oxide. A short-acting neuromuscular blocker (e.g., succinylcholine or mivacurium) is added only if the trachea is to be intubated. Maintenance is usually a balanced technique using sevoflurane or desflurane in oxygen with or without nitrous oxide, small to moderate doses of narcotics, and neuromuscular blockers only when necessary. Resuming spontaneous ventilation before the end of surgery, whenever possible, is preferred so that narcotic can be effectively titrated and overdosing inhalation agent is minimized.

The choices for airway management have increased as technology has expanded to meet our special needs. Often the patient does not need endotracheal intubation if they are fully fasted and have minimal physiologic derangement. Thus a general anesthetic can be managed with a natural airway, as in the case of face-lifts when oxygen may not be used because of concurrent electrocautery. Other options include the cuffed oropharyngeal airway (COPA) and the laryngeal mask airway (LMA), which are supraglottic airway devices that serve as stents to keep the airway patent and conduits through which we can deliver and scavenge volatile anesthetics. They serve a similar function to a mask airway but allow the anesthesiologist a hands-free alternative. An LMA or COPA are useful when one wishes to use a volatile anesthetic but a cuffed endotracheal tube is not required to protect the airway or provide for positive-pressure ventilation.

Management of the anesthetic also includes the intraoperative consideration and treatment of the most common postoperative issues in ambulatory medicine, notably pain and postoperative nausea and vomiting (PONV). PONV and pain are the two leading causes of delay in recovery and unanticipated admission to the hospital. For this reason significant time, resources, and research have been devoted to these two issues.

Pain is best treated preemptively, first and foremost by decreasing anxiety and relieving the patient's concern that their pain will be treated effectively, sufficiently, and in a timely manner. Second, whenever possible, we can perform a preemptive block, i.e., blocking or altering the pain pathways before the noxious surgical stimulus has begun. If intravenous narcotics are to be used they should be given in a dose sufficient to provide analgesia for the entire duration of the surgical procedure and postanesthesia recovery period. Otherwise, the need to administer bolus pain medications in the recovery unit may lead to additional sedation that could delay the patient's discharge from the ambulatory surgery unit. Whenever possible, the surgeon should perform a field block or infuse local anesthesia directly into the wound. When this is done before the surgical incision it is termed "preemptive analgesia" and, allows the anesthesiologist to use minimal narcotics. Use of nonsteroidal anti-inflammatory drugs (NSAIDs, e.g., ketorolac) preoperatively or intraoperatively may decrease or obviate the need for narcotics. Too much or too little pain control can lead to nausea and vomiting, so it is very important to address this issue early and titrate medications to the patient's needs.

Nausea and vomiting are so ubiquitous and multifactorial that we are unable to adequately prevent their occurrence routinely. They occur in 5% to 35% of ambulatory surgical patients despite attempts at minimizing their occurrence, forcing us to admit that there still are no magic bullets to prevent PONV. Many risk factors for PONV exist including preoperative anxiety, dehydration, female sex, pain, high-risk surgeries, intraoperative use of nitrous oxide, history of motion sickness, selection of hypnotic agent, history of previous PONV, and reversal of neuromuscular blockers to name the top 10 risks. For this reason there is no one therapy to prevent or treat PONV, and the best prevention is still hotly debated at national ambulatory anesthesia meetings. The following list is a set of guidelines that we strive to provide for most of our high-risk patients in an effort to decrease this major cause of patient discomfort and delayed recovery.

1. Decrease preoperative anxiety with verbal or pharmacologic anxiolysis, which can best be accomplished at the preoperative interview when possible.
2. Use antiemetics preoperatively or intraoperatively.
3. Perform induction with propofol, and perhaps administer another small dose of propofol as an antiemetic just before emergence.
4. Ensure adequate rehydration.
5. Minimize narcotic analgesia, maximize local anesthetics; use NSAIDs.
6. Avoid reversal of neuromuscular blockers; use shorter-acting neuromuscular blockers or, when possible, none at all.
7. Avoid use of nitrous oxide in high-risk patients.

SUMMARY

Ambulatory anesthesia is a rewarding subspecialty despite its "fast and furious" lifestyle. Outpatient procedures have become the most common type of surgery in this country, and advances in pharmacology and surgical technology have allowed us to increase patient safety and satisfaction. The challenge is to perfect the art of medicine, so that patients having ambulatory surgery do not feel as if they have been given a "factory finish." Every patient must be evaluated, prepared for surgery, anesthetized, and allowed to recover in an efficient but compassionate manner. Despite the sheer volume of cases, the patient must first be treated as an individual.

SUGGESTED READINGS

Wetchler BV. Outpatient anesthesia. In: Stoelting RK, Barash PG, Cullen BF, eds. Clinical Anesthesia. 2nd Ed. Philadelphia: JB Lippincott, 1992:1389–1416.

Henderson JA. Ambulatory surgery: past, present, and future. In: Wetchler BV, ed. Anesthesia for Ambulatory Surgery. 2nd Ed. Philadelphia: JB Lippincott, 1991:1-27.

Gold BS, Kitz DS, Lecky JH, Neuhaus JM. Unanticipated admission to the hospital following ambulatory surgery. JAMA 1989;262:3008–3010.

Watcha MF, White PF. Postoperative nausea and vomiting: its etiology, treatment and prevention. Anesthesiology 1992;77:162–184.

Chung F. Recovery pattern and home-readiness after ambulatory surgery. Anesth Analg 1995;80:896–902.

CHAPTER 15

Anesthesia for Cardiac Surgery

Daniel Talmor, MD, and John S. Mashikian, MD

INTRODUCTION

The practice of anesthesia for cardiac surgery requires the use of skills both as physician and leader of a multidisciplinary team. Currently, coronary artery bypass grafting (CABG) makes up approximately 60% of all cardiac surgeries performed in the United States. In this chapter we will use the example of an adult CABG operation to walk the reader through a typical procedure.

PREOPERATIVE EVALUATION

As with all anesthetics, the care of the patient begins with a comprehensive preoperative evaluation. For the patient undergoing cardiac surgery, this evaluation will need to address a number of issues specific to the cardiac patient.

History and Physical Examination

In addition to a standard anesthetic preoperative evaluation (see Chapter 8), we must address a number of issues with particular relevance to cardiac surgical procedures. Anginal symptoms such as chest pain or tightness with or without radiation to the neck, throat, or arm, epigastric distress, diaphoresis, and other symptoms should be noted and assessed for frequency, duration, and precipitating and relieving factors. Of particular concern are signs and symptoms of acute or chronic heart failure such as paroxysmal nocturnal dyspnea, orthopnea, peripheral edema, and rales on chest auscultation. Obtaining this information will allow the team to optimize the patient's medical status before surgery, which may reduce perioperative morbidity and mortality.

Coexisting pulmonary disease is common in these patients because of the prevalence of cigarette smoking. Signs and symptoms of chronic obstructive pulmonary disease, with or without bronchospasm, are important to note.

Previous chest surgery may complicate the surgical procedure and lead to increased operative time and blood loss. Vascular surgery to the lower extremities may cause problems with vein harvesting or interfere with intra-aortic balloon pump placement if needed.

A thorough history of bleeding diathesis is paramount. Controlled anticoagulation with heparin must be achieved to prevent clotting in the cardiopulmonary bypass (CPB) circuit and to prevent subsequent activation of the fibrinolytic pathway. Patients with preexisting abnormalities of clotting (either as a result of drug therapy, liver disease, or congenital defects) are more likely to suffer from coagulopathy in the post-CPB period, and it is extremely important to define the nature of this abnormality so that appropriate blood product component therapy can be implemented.

Preexisting renal dysfunction increases the likelihood of post-CPB renal failure, which is associated with a perioperative mortality of up to 25% to 50%. Neurologic status must be assessed, with particular attention to previous stroke, transient ischemic attack, and carotid artery disease.

Finally, the patient's medications must be reviewed and a plan for perioperative dosing formulated. In particular, diabetic patients taking insulin or oral hypoglycemic agents must have their regimens modified to take into account reduced glucose intake in the perioperative period, as well as catecholamine-induced perioperative hyperglycemia. Antianginal and antihypertensive medications such as nitrates, β-blockers, calcium-channel blockers, and angiotensin-converting enzyme inhibitors are continued throughout the perioperative period. Antiplatelet medications other than aspirin are typically discontinued. Of course, any drug sensitivities should be noted.

Laboratory Studies

Patients undergoing cardiac surgery require an extensive laboratory evaluation before surgery. Typical laboratory tests performed include a complete blood count for hemoglobin, platelet count, and white blood cell count; chemistry analysis for sodium, potassium, chloride, serum bicarbonate, blood urea nitrogen, and creatinine; serum glucose; liver function tests; and coagulation profile with activated partial thromboplastin time and prothrombin time. Any abnormalities in these studies will guide the need for further analysis. A blood sample for typing and crossmatching blood products is needed.

Electrocardiogram

A 12-lead electrocardiogram (ECG), including a rhythm strip, should be obtained for all patients. Particular attention should be given to evidence of myocardial ischemia (ST-segment or T-wave changes) and conduction defects including bundle branch block. Other important findings may include left or right ventricular hypertrophy, atrial or ventricular ectopy, and evidence of drug or metabolic abnormalities.

Chest Radiograph

Signs of cardiac failure (such as pulmonary edema) and cardiomegaly (defined as a cardiothoracic ratio of >50%) are important findings that may indicate impaired ventricular function. Hyperinflation of lungs indicative of chronic pulmonary disease such as emphysema, consolidations indicative of pneumonia, and interstitial lung disease should be noted.

Echocardiography

Ultrasonographic examination of the heart (echocardiography) has revolutionized the noninvasive evaluation of heart disease, both preoperatively as well as intraoperatively. Overall left and right ventricular function and regional wall motion abnormalities, as well as valvular function, intracardiac defects, cardiomyopathies, pericardial disease, and aortic pathology, may all be diagnosed and quantified by echocardiography.

Stress Testing

Patients undergoing CABG surgery will frequently have undergone a preoperative stress test. Physical exercise on a treadmill stresses the heart while the patient is monitored either by ECG or echocardiography. Areas of myocardium that have a limited blood supply will be exposed by ST-segment changes on ECG or decreased wall thickening on echocardiography. Alternatively, for patients who cannot exercise, the heart is stressed pharmacologically, typically with dobutamine, and then examined with echocardiography. Coronary vasodilators, such as dipyridamole, may also expose areas of myocardium with limited blood flow. This information is useful to the anesthesiologist so that particular areas of myocardium at risk can be closely monitored in the perioperative period.

Cardiac Catheterization

All patients undergoing CABG will have a preoperative cardiac catheterization, which provides both anatomic and functional data. Coronary artery angiography will define the coronary anatomy and quantify any stenoses present and the nature of collateral flow. Significant stenosis is defined as a narrowing of 70% or more, or 50% or greater in the left main coronary artery. A left ventriculogram, in which radiopaque dye is instilled into the left ventricle, will demonstrate wall motion abnormalities and overall left ventricular systolic function, i.e., the ejection fraction (normally greater than 55%). Mitral regurgitation, left ventricular outflow tract abnormalities, and intracardiac shunts may also be appreciated. Measurement of intracardiac pressures during right and left heart catheterization allows for the assessment of pulmonary hypertension and volume status (preload). Left ventricular end-diastolic pressure will be elevated in patients with either volume or pressure overload of the left ventricle. This may be a result of left ventricular failure, volume overload, or poor ventricular compliance owing to myocardial ischemia or hypertrophy. Finally, cardiac catheterization will identify cardiomyopathies and pericardial disease.

PREMEDICATION

The most effective way to reduce perioperative patient anxiety is a thoughtful and thorough preoperative visit by the anesthesiologist during which all patient concerns are addressed and answered completely. In addition premedication is usually given the night before and the morning of surgery and usually consists of a benzodiazepine (e.g., midazolam) for anxiolysis and amnesia, with or without a narcotic (e.g., morphine) for analgesia. If needed, these drugs may be supplemented in the preoperative holding area during line placement. All premedicated patients should receive supplemental oxygen by face mask to minimize hypoxia caused by respiratory depression.

PATIENT MONITORING

In addition to the standard monitors used during anesthesia (see Chapter 6), patients undergoing cardiac surgery require additional more-complex and invasive monitoring.

Electrocardiography

A five-lead ECG system allows for monitoring of seven ECG leads: three bipolar limb leads (I, II, III), three augmented limb leads (aVR, aVL, aVF), and one of six unipolar precordial leads (V_1 through V_6). The use of auto-mated, real-time ST-segment analysis has been shown to increase the sensitivity of ischemia monitoring by ECG. Lead II should always be one of the leads monitored because its vector orientation parallels that of atrial depolarization, and it is therefore the best lead for determining rhythm. Simultaneous monitoring of leads II and V_5 has been reported to detect 80% of ischemic events.

Temperature Monitoring

Most cardiac surgeries are performed with some degree of hypothermia. This reduces total body (including myocardial) oxygen consumption, an important protective mechanism during periods of reduced flow. Ideally two temperatures should be monitored. Central (or core) temperature is usually monitored in the nasopharynx, rectum, pulmonary artery, or urinary bladder. Peripheral temperature can be monitored with a skin or forehead probe. During rewarming of the patient after CPB it is not unusual to see large differences between the central and peripheral temperatures. Failure to rewarm the periphery adequately may lead to postoperative hypothermia when the two compartments equilibrate.

Urinary Catheter

Urine output is an excellent indirect monitor of systemic perfusion and intravascular volume status. Additionally, a catheter protects the bladder from overdistension and can provide a means to monitor temperature, as discussed above.

Arterial Blood Pressure Monitoring

Continuous monitoring of arterial blood pressure from a peripheral artery is essential during cardiac surgery. The radial artery is typically used, but other possibilities include femoral, brachial, and axillary arteries. Arterial cannulation also allows sampling for arterial blood gas analysis (pH, Po_2, and Pco_2), glucose, and electrolytes.

Intravenous Access

All patients having cardiac surgery require both peripheral and central venous access. Peripheral access usually consists of one or two large-bore (14 or 16-gauge) catheters placed in one or both of the upper extremities and is the primary means by which fluid and blood products will be given. After transport of the patient to the operating room and instituting monitoring of ECG, arterial blood pressure, and pulse oximetry, the anesthesiologist will then proceed to obtain central access. Catheterization of a central vein is important for measuring central venous pressure (CVP) and for the administration of anesthetic and vasoactive drugs. Most stable patients with normal ventricular function and without significant valvular, pulmonary, or renal disease may be safely monitored using only a CVP line.

Pulmonary Artery Catheter

Patients with decreased ventricular function, unstable conditions, significant valvular disease, or significant comorbid conditions usually have a pulmonary artery catheter (PAC) placed. The advantages of a PAC include more-accurate measurement of intravascular volume (preload) and a means of measuring cardiac output with subsequent calculation of stroke volume and both systemic and pulmonary vascular resistances. These measurements will be especially useful during separation from CPB and in the postoperative period. In addition, specialized PACs are available with cardiac pacing capability and continuous measurement of cardiac output and pulmonary artery oxygen saturation.

Transesophageal Echocardiography

A relatively recent development has been the routine use of intraoperative monitoring by transesophageal echocardiography (TEE). Although it is possible to see the right side of the heart during surgery, and a PAC gives us indirect indices of left ventricular function, TEE allows for a direct, real-time analysis of cardiac function. Uses of TEE include evaluation of both left and right ventricular function; determination of valvular anatomy and function; ischemia monitoring; detection of aortic plaque or intracardiac thrombi, air, and shunts; assessment of the adequacy of surgical repair and revascularization; and monitoring of intravascular volume status. TEE can also be used to guide the placement of various catheters, intra-aortic balloon pumps, and ventricular-assist devices. The TEE probe is placed after induction of anesthesia. A full examination of the heart and great vessels is performed in the pre-CPB period, with particular attention to each patient's specific condition and indication for surgery. This will allow detection of any unanticipated anomalies and provide a baseline with which the post-CPB examination can be compared.

COURSE OF THE PROCEDURE

The CABG procedure can be divided into three broad stages on the basis of the relationship to CPB: the pre-CPB period including anesthetic induction, CPB, and the post-CPB period. Each period has its unique considerations.

Pre-CPB

The major goal of the cardiac anesthesiologist during this time is to induce general anesthesia and prevent further insult to the heart before the patient undergoes CPB while the bypass grafts are constructed. Paramount in this effort is the preservation of the relationship between myocardial oxygen supply and demand. This is determined by the content of oxygen in blood, the amount of blood circulated to the heart, and the quantity of oxygen extracted by the heart. Myocardial oxygen supply is maintained by providing adequate oxygen saturation of the blood, hemoglobin level, and cardiac output. In addition, coronary perfusion pressure, defined as the difference between mean aortic diastolic pressure and left ventricular diastolic pressure, must also be maintained. Compromise of the coronary circulation by either thrombosis or narrowing of the epicardial vessels will also reduce the delivery of oxygen to the heart. Myocardial oxygen demand must also be limited by manipulating heart rate, contractility, and wall tension. Any imbalance of this relationship, either by a decrease in oxygen supply, or an increase in oxygen demand, may lead to myocardial ischemia and potentially irreversible myocardial damage.

Preoperative left ventricular function is a major consideration when choosing an anesthetic technique. Patients with poor left ventricular function will not tolerate what otherwise may be considered appropriate anesthetic agents. On the other hand, patients with preserved ventricular function will often show an impressive sympathetic response to intubation, resulting in considerable hypertension and tachycardia. Either response will result in a worsening of the myocardial oxygen supply to demand ratio and may lead to myocardial ischemia.

INDUCTION OF ANESTHESIA

After placement of peripheral intravenous lines and arterial cannula in the holding area, the patient is brought to the operating room where ECG and pulse oximetry monitoring is instituted. Central venous access is typically obtained after the patient has general anesthesia induced. The patient is preoxygenated with 100% oxygen for 3 to 5 minutes. Induction of general anesthesia is typically accomplished with a combination of narcotic (fentanyl), barbiturate (sodium thiopental), and inhalation agent such as isoflurane. Mask ventilation is established, and neuromuscular blocking agent (pancuronium) is given to facilitate endotracheal intubation.

Traditionally, a high-dose narcotic technique has been used to induce general anesthesia for cardiac surgery because narcotics provide the most hemodynamically stable conditions for laryngoscopy and intubation. This technique involves giving as much as 25 to 50 μg/kg fentanyl (or equipotent dose of other narcotic) for induction. In the past decade it was realized that a more traditional "balanced" technique can be used with equal hemodynamic stability. This technique involves giving a lower dose of narcotic (5 to 15 μg/kg fentanyl) combined with a modest dose of sodium thiopental (2 to 4 mg/kg) and supplemental isoflurane. The lower narcotic dose technique offers the advantage of earlier emergence from anesthesia at the conclusion of the surgery.

Before laryngoscopy and intubation, the patient's response to a series of graded stimulations is observed. An oral airway is placed, followed by catheterization of the urinary bladder. If there is no evidence of sympathetic response (e.g., increases in heart rate or blood pressure), laryngoscopy and endotracheal intubation are performed. If a sympathetic response is observed, then supplemental narcotic is given or the inspired concentration of isoflurane is increased until the response is blunted. Maintenance of anesthesia is accomplished with additional doses of narcotic, benzodiazepines, isoflurane, and neuromuscular blocker. It is not uncommon for the patient to become mildly hypotensive in the period between anesthetic induction and the start of surgery as a result of the vasodilatory action of the anesthetic agents. At this time, blood pressure is typically maintained with small boluses or infusion of phenylephrine, an α-adrenergic agonist.

PREPARATION FOR CARDIOPULMONARY BYPASS

After induction of anesthesia the patient is prepped and draped, and the surgery is begun. The surgeons will open the chest via median sternotomy, dissect the left internal mammary artery, and perform the arterial and venous cannulations necessary to perform CPB. Simultaneously, the saphenous vein is harvested from the leg. Various degrees of stimulation and sympathetic response characterize each of these stages. It is imperative that the anesthesiologist be aware of times of maximal stimulation so that anesthetic depth can be adjusted to prevent a sympathetic response and possible disruption of the myocardial oxygen supply-demand relationship. Times of increased stimulation include surgical incision, sternotomy, pericardiotomy, and aortic cannulation. It is imperative that a high index of suspicion be maintained for the occurrence of myocardial ischemia as evidenced by ECG changes, elevation of pulmonary artery pressures, wall motion abnormalities on TEE, or hemodynamic instability.

MANAGEMENT OF MYOCARDIAL ISCHEMIA

If any myocardial ischemia is detected, appropriate action must be taken to avoid or limit myocardial damage. The measures that are taken are determined by the mechanism of the ischemia, and this is determined by the various monitors that we use. Tachycardia and hypercontractility are treated with β-blockers or calcium-channel blockers; increased wall tension or vasospasm, with nitroglycerin; suspected thrombosis, with anticoagulation with heparin; anemia, with packed red blood cells; hypoxia, with increased inspired fraction of oxygen or change in mechanical ventilation; hypotension, with vasopressors such as phenylephrine; and decreased myocardial systolic function, with inotropic agents. Frequently the exact cause of the ischemia is not readily apparent, and a variety of measures are instituted simultaneously.

ANTICOAGULATION

In preparation for instituting CPB, it is necessary to achieve adequate anticoagulation inasmuch as the entire CPB circuit is thrombogenic. Inadequate anticoagulation may result in overt thrombus in the bypass circuit, or more subtly, microthrombus formation and stimulation of the fibrinolytic system resulting in post-CPB bleeding. Anticoagulation is achieved with heparin, in doses from 3 to 4 mg/kg. (One milligram of heparin is equivalent to 100 U of activity.) Anticoagulation is monitored with the activated clotting time (ACT). The ACT is a modification of the whole blood clotting time wherein a blood sample is added to a test tube containing a surface activator (typically diatomaceous earth). Adequate anticoagulation for CPB is generally thought to be an ACT greater than 400 seconds.

Cardiopulmonary Bypass

The goal of CPB is to separate the central (cardiopulmonary) and systemic circulations so that the heart can be arrested and the rest of the body and brain can still be perfused. The combination of CPB and myocardial standstill creates a bloodless, motionless surgical field, which optimizes operating conditions during construction of the epicardial coronary artery bypass grafts. Blood is drained (either by gravity or with vacuum assistance) from the patient's right atrium or femoral vein and collected in a reservoir on the bypass machine. It is then pumped through an oxygenator in which the blood is oxygenated and carbon dioxide is removed (Fig. 15-1). The perfusionist controls both the fraction of inspired oxygen and the rate of oxygen flow through the membrane, thereby controlling the patient's arterial oxygen and carbon dioxide levels, respectively. The treated blood then passes through an air filter and is returned to the patient via an arterial cannula placed either in the patient's ascending aorta or femoral artery. The amount of blood flow provided to the patient (i.e., the cardiac output) is also controlled by the perfusionist. Mild to moderate systemic hypothermia ($28°$ to $34°C$) is used during bypass to minimize oxygen consumption of both the body and brain.

After CPB is established, an aortic cross-clamp is applied to the ascending aorta between the aortic cannula and the patient's heart. The time during which the cross-clamp remains in place is referred to as the ischemic time, because no blood is allowed to enter the coronary arteries. The heart is then arrested by delivering a high-concentration potassium solution (called cardioplegia) down the native coronary arteries (antegrade cardio-

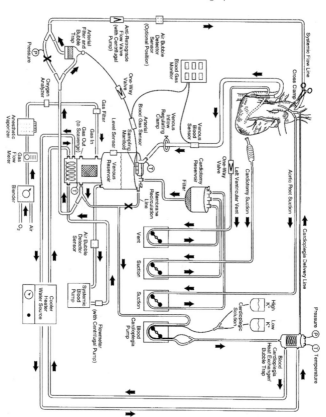

FIGURE 15-1. Cardiopulmonary bypass circuit. (Adapted with permission from Gravlee GP, Davis RF, Kurusz M, Utley JR, eds. Cardiopulmonary Bypass: Principles and Practices. 2nd Ed. Baltimore: Lippincott Williams & Wilkins, 2000:70.)

plegia) via a cannula placed between the aortic cross-clamp and the heart. Cardioplegia is also given backwards through the venous system of the myocardium (retrograde cardioplegia) via a catheter placed in the coronary sinus. Potassium is used as the arresting agent because it will arrest the heart in diastole and thus minimize oxygen consumption. During CPB, the perfusionist draws blood samples to monitor the patient's arterial pH, oxygen, carbon dioxide, potassium, and glucose levels.

MYOCARDIAL PROTECTION

Several measures are taken to protect the heart during ischemic time because irreversible myocardial damage may otherwise occur. Electromechanical arrest is the most important protective measure as the beating action of the heart accounts for approximately 85% of the heart's total oxygen consumption. The heart is cooled to approximately 10°C with cold cardioplegia solution (4°C) and supplemented with topical ice slush. Additionally, the left ventricle is vented to prevent its distension, which may lead to subendocardial ischemia. Finally, various additives are included in the cardioplegia solution to minimize myocardial edema, maintain normal intramyocardial pH, and provide substrate for anaerobic metabolism.

MAINTENANCE OF ANESTHESIA

During the mild hypothermia of CPB the patient's anesthetic requirement is diminished but not eliminated. Small doses of benzodiazepines or narcotics are typically given to the patient intravenously, which the perfusionist can supplement with isoflurane added to the bypass machine. It is important to give neuromuscular blockers before instituting bypass not only to prevent the patient from moving during this time but, more importantly, to prevent subtle shivering that may occur with hypothermia, which can lead to muscle breakdown, myoglobinuria, and possibly renal damage.

WEANING FROM CARDIOPULMONARY BYPASS

Weaning from CPB is the process during which the patient's own cardiopulmonary function is restored. During this time the patient's body temperature is returned to normal by a heater on the bypass machine. The aortic cross-clamp is removed, allowing blood to reperfuse the heart and wash out any residual cardioplegia solution, and any metabolic derangements are corrected. While the heart is reperfused it is not uncommon for ventricular fibrillation to occur, which is promptly treated with a defibrillating countershock applied directly to the myocardium. The surgeon places atrial and ventricular epicardial pacing wires so that the heart can be externally paced if needed. Normal sinus rhythm at 80 to 90 beats per minute is optimal. Hemodynamic control is usually shared by the perfusionist and the anesthesiologist at this time, such that the perfusionist controls the patient's cardiac output via the bypass machine and the anesthesiologist controls the blood pressure by manipulating vascular tone with either vasoconstricting agents (e.g., phenylephrine, norepinephrine) or vasodilating drugs (e.g., nitroglycerin, nitroprusside, isoflurane).

The goal of treatment is a cardiac index greater than 2 L/min/m² of body surface area and a mean arterial pressure between 50 and 60 mm Hg.

The patient's lungs are reinflated, and mechanical ventilation is resumed by the anesthesiologist. The patient's blood is then gradually returned from the bypass machine to the patient, and the heart is allowed to resume its usual pumping function. The processes of oxygenation, ventilation, and cardiac function are once again the responsibility of the anesthesiologist.

HEMODYNAMIC SUPPORT

Most patients will have adequate myocardial function after CPB and will not require an inotropic agent (e.g., dobutamine, epinephrine, milrinone) to support the circulation. Exceptions to this may be patients with poor preoperative ventricular function, uncorrected valvular disease, or inadequate myocardial protection or revascularization during bypass. The optimal inotropic drug is a matter of considerable debate, with no clear evidence in favor of any particular drug. Determining the type of hemodynamic support required is based on data obtained from the PAC, TEE, and direct observation of the heart.

Post-CPB

After successful separation from bypass two major issues that confront the anesthesiologist are the maintenance of hemodynamic stability and the normalization of coagulation. The hemodynamic goals are essentially the same as those in the pre-CPB period: maintenance of adequate systemic perfusion, ensuring a balance between myocardial oxygen supply and demand, and avoidance of myocardial ischemia. These goals are met by continuing the pharmacologic support begun before separation from bypass and modifying the drug regimen as necessary. Continuous monitoring of arterial blood pressure, cardiac filling pressures, stroke volume, and contractility (as determined by PAC and TEE) will guide this therapy.

COAGULOPATHY

After weaning from CPB, and before the surgeon decannulates the heart and closes the chest, it is necessary to normalize the patient's coagulation status. Protamine is given to neutralize any residual heparin, and dosing can be based on the patient's weight, total amount of heparin given, or assay of residual heparin activity as determined by ACT. Institutional preference governs which technique is used inasmuch as all have proven effective. Several adverse responses to protamine administration are possible and include histamine-induced systemic hypotension, IgE-mediated allergic reactions, and complement-mediated catastrophic pulmonary hypertension.

In addition to heparin-associated coagulopathy, other clotting abnormalities are possible, most of which result either directly or indirectly from the use of CPB. The tubing, reservoir, and oxygenator membrane are all foreign bodies that serve to activate the clotting cascade. Because the pump must be primed with either normal saline or lactated Ringer's solution, there is a significant dilutional effect on all blood components, most importantly red cells, platelets, and clotting factors. Both quantitative and qualitative derangements must be diagnosed and treated, possibly requiring transfusion of platelets, fresh-frozen plasma, or cryoprecipitate.

CHEST CLOSURE

After both the aortic and venous cannulas have been removed and adequate hemostasis has been achieved, the sternal edges are brought together and secured with titanium wires. Significant hemodynamic decompensation may occur at this time as a result of compression of the heart and great vessels, deformation of the newly constructed bypass grafts, or compromised venous return. The right ventricle is particularly susceptible during chest closure, and signs of right heart failure must be closely monitored. Once the sternum is closed, the patient's arterial blood pressure, CVP, and pulmonary artery pressures should be compared with their previous values. If a PAC is used, cardiac output should be determined. TEE is extremely useful in this situation to help diagnose the cause of any hemodynamic changes. After chest closure, confirmation of hemodynamic stability, and adequate medical and surgical hemostasis, the patient may be transferred to the intensive care unit. After cardiac surgery, patients are generally not awakened and extubated in the operating room. Instead, they are extubated after one to several hours in the intensive care unit.

TRANSPORT TO THE INTENSIVE CARE UNIT

Transporting a critically ill patient is a potentially dangerous process and requires extreme vigilance by the anesthesiologist. During transport, just as in the operating room, the patient is continuously monitored, including arterial blood pressure, pulmonary artery pressure or CVP, ECG, and pulse oximetry. The TEE probe is removed just before transferring the patient from the operating room table to the transport bed, which should be equipped with a full oxygen tank, ambu bag and mask, intubation equipment, resuscitation drugs, and a defibrillator. Infusions of vasoactive drugs (if used) must continue without interruption during transport to the intensive care unit.

SUMMARY

Although it is beyond the scope of this chapter to discuss all of the different types of cardiac surgery, each with their particular anesthetic concerns, many of the principles described above can be applied to all cases. In particular, a complete and thorough preoperative evaluation is always indicated and is of paramount importance in developing a comprehensive and safe anesthetic plan. The principles involving CPB are the same whether the patient is undergoing a revascularization procedure, valve repair or replacement, or correction of a congenital defect.

SUGGESTED READINGS

DiNardo JA. Anesthesia for Cardiac Surgery. 2nd Ed. Stamford, Conn.: Appleton & Lange, 1998.

Kaplan JA. Cardiac Anesthesia. 3rd Ed. Philadelphia: WB Saunders, 1993.

CHAPTER 16

Obstetric Anesthesia

Stephen Pratt, MD

INTRODUCTION

Care of the pregnant patient presents distinctive challenges to the obstetric anesthesiologist who must consider the physiologic changes of pregnancy, concerns for the well-being of the fetus (the second patient), and the impact of various pregnancy-related conditions. With cesarean section rates climbing well above 20% nationally, and requests for labor epidural analgesia approaching 90% in some centers, anesthesiologists care for an ever-increasing number of pregnant women. Not only is it incumbent on all anesthesiologists to understand how to best care for these patients, but all physicians should be familiar with the physiology and management of this population.

PHYSIOLOGIC CHANGES OF PREGNANCY

Pregnancy causes changes in every major organ system. These changes begin early in pregnancy and progress throughout gestation. The anesthesiologist must understand these changes to diagnose and properly treat pathologic conditions, and to safely conduct anesthesia in the pregnant patient.

Cardiovascular System

Maternal metabolic requirements and oxygen consumption progressively increase throughout pregnancy. By term, oxygen consumption has increased 20% or more. Metabolic requirements increase approximately 14%. Both the cardiovascular and respiratory systems must adapt to meet these changes, and to prepare the mother for the stress of labor. The cardiovascular changes of pregnancy are outlined in Table 16-1.

Aortocaval Compression

In 1953, Howard described a syndrome of maternal hypotension, tachycardia, and an increase in femoral venous pressure associated with the supine position. He postulated that this was caused by compression of the inferior vena cava (IVC) by the gravid uterus. It is now recognized that IVC compression occurs in nearly all term pregnant women who lie supine.

Aortocaval compression syndrome can occur without evidence of maternal hypotension, however. Pressure from the gravid uterus on the abdominal aorta can increase proximal arterial resistance and thus may actually increase brachial artery blood pressure. However, femoral (and thus uterine) artery hypotension may occur. The increase in femoral venous

Table 16-1. Cardiovascular and Respiratory Changes of Pregnancy

Cardiovascular Changes		Respiratory Changes	
Variable	*% Change*	*Variable*	*% Change*
Heart rate	↑ 15%–30%	Total lung capacity	↓ 0%–5%
Systolic blood pressure	↑ 0%–8%	Forced vital capacity	0%
Diastolic blood pressure	↓ 0%–20%	Tidal volume	↑ 25%–45%
Mean arterial pressure	↓ 0%–15%	Functional residual capacity	↓ 10%–25%
Cardiac output	↑ 35%–60%	Expiratory reserve volume	↓ 10%–40%
Stroke volume	↑ 13%–33%	Residual volume	↓ 0%–20%
Central venous pressure	↔	FEV_1	0%
Pulmonary capillary wedge pressure	↔ or slight ↓	Minute ventilation	↑ 20%–50%
Systemic vascular resistance	↓ 20%-35%	Alveolar ventilation	↑ 60%–70%
Pulmonary vascular resistance	↓ 34%	Dead space	↑ 24%
Red blood cell mass	↑ 20%	Respiratory rate	↔
Plasma volume	↑ 45%	Oxygen consumption	↑ 18%–33%
Blood volume	↑ 44%-50%	CO_2 production	↑ 30%–40%

FEV_1, forced expiratory volume in 1 second.

pressure further decreases uterine perfusion pressure, leading to fetal compromise.

Prevention of aortocaval compression is paramount. Beginning at approximately 20 weeks gestation, the pregnant woman should not lie supine. Placing a wedge under the right hip or tipping the operating table to create a 15% leftward tilt will relieve the compression in most women. However, this maneuver is not 100% effective, and the anesthesiologist must be ever vigilant for signs of maternal or fetal compromise.

Respiratory System

Capillary engorgement and mucosal edema of the upper airway are common at term. This can produce nasal obstruction and epistaxis. Laryngeal edema may cause voice changes and has even caused upper airway obstruction. The expanding uterus causes an elevation of the diaphragm and an increase in both the anteroposterior and transverse diameters of the thorax. Diaphragmatic excursion is unaffected by this cephalad shift. Mild dyspnea is common at term, and may make the diagnosis of cardiopulmonary disease more difficult.

Progesterone is a respiratory stimulant that produces an increase in respiratory rate early in pregnancy. Later, as CO_2 production increases there is an additional rise in minute ventilation. The relative hyperventilation of pregnancy decreases arterial P_{CO_2} to 27 to 34 mm Hg. Arterial P_{O_2} increases to 106 to 108 mm Hg in early pregnancy, but falls slightly in the third trimester. Table 16-1 outlines the respiratory changes associated with pregnancy.

Uterus and Placenta

The placenta is a large disk-shaped organ derived from both maternal and fetal tissues. It acts as the fetal respiratory, excretory, and gastrointestinal systems. Because surgery and anesthesia can cause alterations in uteroplacental function, an understanding of this organ is essential.

Uterine blood flow may be 700 mL/min or more (up to 10% of maternal cardiac output). The uterine vessels have limited ability to autoregulate, which means that uterine blood flow (and therefore fetal nutrient delivery) is dependent on perfusion pressure. The uterine vessels ultimately give rise to spiral arteries that pierce the basal plate of the placenta and circulate blood into the intervillous space. The maternal blood then returns through the basal plate. Two umbilical arteries deliver fetal blood to the placenta. They eventually divide into capillaries that traverse the placental villi. These villi project into the intervillous space, are bathed by maternal blood, and are the unit of nutrient exchange. Blood returns to the fetus through a single umbilical vein.

The placenta also has important synthetic and metabolic functions. It is the primary source of the hormones necessary to maintain pregnancy. It may serve as a filter of sorts, metabolizing unwanted substances before they can reach the fetus.

Most anesthetic agents readily cross the placenta and enter the fetal circulation (neuromuscular blocking agents are an exception because they are large, charged molecules that do not readily cross lipid membranes). Despite this, most newborns are not significantly depressed by anesthetic medications, even when born while the mother is under general anesthesia. Metabolism by the fetal liver may account for this. As blood returns to the fetus in the umbilical vein, it traverses the liver via the ductus venosus. Up to 75% of this blood enters the substrate of the liver and is therefore subject to metabolism.

Other Changes

GASTROINTESTINAL

The expanding uterus exerts increasing pressure on the abdominal viscera, thus intragastric pressure increases throughout gestation. In addition, progesterone decreases lower esophageal sphincter tone in many women, leading to a high (up to 80%) incidence of gastroesophageal reflux. Gastric emptying is dramatically delayed during labor and does not return to normal for 24 to 48 hours after delivery. Older studies indicated that gastric emptying was delayed throughout pregnancy, beginning as early as 8 to 12 weeks of gestation. More recent work refutes these data.

ENDOCRINE

Pregnancy has been described as a diabetogenic state, characterized by an increase in basal hepatic glucose production and relative insulin resistance in late pregnancy. Despite this, there is usually a fall in maternal serum glucose concentration throughout gestation. Increased maternal blood volume and a greater insulin response to a meal are likely explanations for this finding. However, up to 4% of pregnancies in the United States are complicated by diabetes (most commonly gestational diabetes).

CENTRAL NERVOUS SYSTEM

Engorgement of the extradural venous plexus leads to a decrease in both the extradural and cerebrospinal fluid (CSF) volumes, and an increased incidence of inadvertent epidural venopuncture during epidural catheter placement (up to 18%).

Pregnant women are more sensitive to the effects of both inhalation and local anesthetics. For example, the minimum alveolar concentration (MAC) of isoflurane is decreased by nearly 33% at term. MAC returns to nonpregnant levels within 72 hours postpartum. Animal and human models demonstrate increased nerve sensitivity to local anesthetics in pregnancy. This appears to be related to the effects of progesterone.

HEMATOLOGIC

Maternal blood volume increases 40% to 50% above nonpregnant values. The increase in plasma volume is greater (40% to 60%) than the increase in red cell mass (approximately 20%), leading to the "physiologic" anemia of pregnancy. Hematocrit values generally decrease to 30% to 35%.

Pregnancy increases the plasma concentration of all clotting factors except factors XI and XIII. The most significant rise occurs in factors VII, VIII, and X, and fibrinogen. There is a rise in serum procoagulants, increased fibrinolytic activity, and an increase in turnover of clotting factors. Conversely, there is a decrease in serum anticoagulants, including antithrombin III and protein S, leading to the hypercoagulable state of pregnancy.

Thrombocytopenia develops in up to 8.3% of gravidas. Incidental thrombocytopenia is the most common cause, with platelet counts rarely falling below 100,000/μL. Other causes include idiopathic thrombocytopenia purpura and the syndrome of hemolysis, elevated liver enzymes, and low platelets (HELLP).

RENAL

During pregnancy, there is an average increase in total body water of more than 8 L. By mid-pregnancy, renal blood flow has increased by 60% to 80%, leading to a 40% to 65% increase in glomerular filtration rate. The glomerulus becomes slightly more permeable to serum proteins, and urinary protein excretion may increase to 500 mg/day.

ANESTHESIA FOR NONOBSTETRIC SURGERY

Whenever possible, elective surgery in the pregnant patient should be delayed until after delivery. This is not always possible, however, and approximately 2% of women (up to 80,000/yr) require surgery during pregnancy. Maternal anesthetic risk is influenced by the altered physiology of pregnancy. Risks to the fetus include potential teratogenic effects of anesthetic medications, hypoxia as a result of alterations in uteroplacental blood flow, and preterm labor.

Maternal Problems Related to Anesthesia

DIFFICULT INTUBATION

Airway edema, maternal weight gain, and breast engorgement contribute to an increased likelihood of difficult or failed intubation. Failed intubation occurs in up to 1 in 250 parturients (which is approximately 10 times higher than the nonpregnant population). Failed and esophageal intubation are leading causes of anesthesia-related maternal deaths.

RAPID DESATURATION

Because of the decreased functional residual capacity (FRC) and increased oxygen consumption, arterial oxygen tension falls three times faster in the pregnant patient than in nonpregnant women. Despite adequate preoxygenation, dangerous arterial desaturation may occur after only 2 to 3 minutes of apnea (compared with 6 to 8 minutes in the general population).

HYPOTENSION

Maternal hypotension is a common and undesirable side effect of anesthesia. The hypotensive effects of general or regional anesthesia combined with aortocaval compression may cause maternal or fetal compromise. Decreased responsiveness to catecholamines can further exacerbate this problem.

ASPIRATION OF GASTRIC CONTENTS

The high incidence of gastroesophageal reflux increases the risk of aspiration during general anesthesia. Other factors (full stomach, emergent or abdominal surgery, difficult intubation) may also contribute to this risk in the pregnant population.

HIGH SPINAL

Increased sensitivity to local anesthetics and the decreased lumbar CSF volume increase the likelihood of high (or even total) spinal anesthetic block. The local anesthetic dose should be decreased in the pregnant patient.

GENERAL ANESTHESIA OVERDOSE

Because of increased sensitivity to inhaled anesthetics, a small FRC, and increased minute ventilation, changes in anesthetic depth occur rapidly in the pregnant patient. Care must be taken to avoid overdose of these agents.

COAGULATION

Pregnancy-related thrombocytopenia may preclude the use of regional anesthesia. Regional anesthesia is considered safe with a platelet count greater than 100,000/mL; its use is controversial when it is between 50,000/mL and 100,000/mL.

FETAL PROBLEMS RELATED TO ANESTHESIA

Fetal concerns in the pregnant surgical patient include potential teratogenic effects of the anesthetics, fetal asphyxia, and preterm labor.

Many commonly used anesthetic agents are teratogens in animals. Because of dramatic interspecies variability, however, the relevance of these data in humans is uncertain. To date, no anesthetic agent has been conclusively shown to cause fetal abnormalities in humans.

However, two agents remain controversial. Chronic maternal exposure to benzodiazepines has been associated with fetal cleft lip and palate. A causal relationship has not been definitively demonstrated, however. Nitrous oxide inhibits methionine synthetase, an enzyme necessary for DNA synthesis. Although there is evidence that inhibition of placental methionine synthetase does occur after only short exposure to nitrous oxide, no data exist to prove that this is associated with fetal abnormalities.

FETAL ASPHYXIA

Fetal oxygenation depends on uterine blood flow (UBF), maternal arterial oxygen content, and the appropriate transfer of maternal oxygen to the fetus. Although anesthetic agents have little direct effect on UBF, anesthesia-induced maternal hypotension may cause it to decrease. Prevention of hypotension, with appropriate medication dosing, adequate prehydration, and left uterine displacement, is the goal. Should maternal hypotension occur, ephedrine (5 to 10 mg intravenously) is the vasopressor of choice as it improves both maternal blood pressure and UBF.

Some authors recommend the use of fetal heart rate (FHR) monitoring during anesthesia to help assess fetal well-being. Changes in the FHR, including decreased heart rate variability or bradycardia, may be early signs of fetal compromise. However, FHR monitoring may be impractical during many procedures. In addition, anesthetic agents decrease FHR variability, making interpretation less reliable.

PRETERM LABOR

Surgery and anesthesia during pregnancy are associated with an increased incidence of both preterm delivery and low birth weight. The overall incidence of prematurity is increased by approximately 50% among pregnant women who have surgery, but it is unclear whether type of anesthesia contributes to the risk of preterm delivery. The incidence of preterm labor appears to be decreased during the second trimester. Whenever possible, uterine activity should be monitored in the postoperative period to detect early signs of labor.

LABOR ANALGESIA

The Nature of Labor Pain

The pain of labor is poorly understood and remarkably variable. Some women describe only mild pain, whereas for others, labor may be the most painful experience of their lives. The mechanism of first-stage labor pain is not well established. Theories include uterine ischemia, activation of cervical stretch receptors, pressure on surrounding pelvic structures, and nerve sensitization from prostaglandins or other chemicals involved in labor. It is visceral in nature, often described as aching, cramping, or burning. First-stage pain is transmitted by the T10 to L2 nerve roots. Generally, first-stage pain is located over the abdomen, but it may radiate to the back, perineum, or legs.

Second-stage pain is caused by pressure on or disruption of pain-sensitive structures in the pelvis, especially the vagina. It is somatic and carried by the S2 to S4 nerve roots.

OPTIONS FOR LABOR ANALGESIA

Nonpharmacologic

In 1951, Lamaze introduced a system of breathing and relaxation techniques designed to reduce the pain and stress of labor. Several years later, Grantly Dick-Read coined the term "natural childbirth." He suggested that labor pain was caused by maternal anxiety and fear, which led to pelvic muscle tension and subsequent pain. He advocated the use of relaxation and breathing techniques to alleviate fear, decrease tension, and minimize pain. The techniques described by these two men remain mainstays of childbirth education today.

Childbirth education, psychoprophylaxis, breathing and relaxation techniques, and emotional support by a friend, family member, or professional (midwife or doula) remain popular. Reported benefits of these techniques include decreased pain, improved maternal satisfaction, shortened labor, and decreased cesarean section rates. Other nonpharmacologic techniques described for labor analgesia include hydrotherapy, massage, transcutaneous electrical nerve stimulation (TENS), biofeedback, hypnosis, and acupuncture or acupressure.

Systemic Medications

Opioid analgesics have become the medications of choice for systemic labor analgesia. Parenteral opioids can be administered by intermittent bolus (intramuscular or intravenous) or by patient-controlled analgesia (PCA). Commonly used medications include morphine, meperidine (Demerol), hydromorphone (Dilaudid), oxymorphone (Numorphan), nalbuphine (Nubain), and butorphanol (Stadol). Recently, patient-controlled techniques have been described using fentanyl and remifentanil. Opioid-based techniques are simple and inexpensive. Disadvantages include relatively poor pain relief and the potential for sedation of both the mother and newborn.

Various tranquilizers may be used as adjuncts to opioid analgesia. Although these medications generally do not possess direct analgesic properties, their sedative and anxiolytic effects may aid relaxation. Commonly used medications include phenothiazines (Phenergan), hydroxyzine (Vistaril), scopolamine, and several barbiturates (secobarbital, amobarbital) and benzodiazepines (midazolam). As with the opiates, these medications can cause respiratory depression in both the mother and the fetus.

Neuraxial Techniques

Lumbar epidural analgesia (LEA) and combined spinal epidural (CSE) are increasingly popular forms of labor analgesia. Some centers report LEA rates approaching 90%. LEA and CSE are safe and very effective when administered by skilled physicians. Major complications are rare, but the anesthesiologist must be trained to take care of them should they occur (see Chapter 5 for a description of the epidural and spinal anesthetic techniques and complications).

Medications

As recently as 20 years ago, large doses of local anesthetics were the mainstay of LEA. Up to 20 mL of 0.5% bupivacaine was frequently administered. This produced a sensory and motor blockade adequate to perform surgery; however, maternal hypotension was common, and complications of local anesthetic toxicity were a significant cause of anesthesia-related maternal morbidity. In addition, the dense sensory and motor block caused some women to feel disconnected from their birth experience. Recently, low-dose epidural techniques have gained popularity.

Pain during the first stage of labor is usually less intense than at later stages. Epidural narcotics alone may provide adequate analgesia in early labor. In addition, the T10 to L2 nerve fibers are small and easily blocked by local anesthetics. The addition of low concentrations of local anesthetics (as low as 0.032% bupivacaine) provides satisfactory analgesia for a majority of women. These ultralow-dose techniques decrease the incidence of side effects. In addition, they allow the parturient to maintain a sense of control during labor and may even permit ambulation.

As labor progresses, pain generally increases. In addition, the sacral roots that transmit the pain of second stage are larger and more resistant to local anesthetic blockade. Although low-dose epidural techniques may continue to provide adequate pain relief throughout labor, some women may require two to three times the initial dose as labor progresses.

Commonly used local anesthetics used for LEA include bupivacaine, lidocaine, ropivacaine, and levo-bupivacaine. Fentanyl and sufentanil are the narcotics administered. Neostigmine and clonidine have been described as adjuncts for LEA, although to date they do not appear to offer any advantages.

Epidural medications can be administered by a continuous infusion, intermittent boluses, or with patient-controlled epidural analgesia (PCEA). The bolus and PCEA techniques are generally associated with lower drug dosage.

The CSE technique has gained widespread popularity in recent years. A small dose of a narcotic (generally fentanyl of sufentanil), often combined with a local anesthetic, is administered into the intrathecal space. This provides satisfactory analgesia for 60 to 150 minutes. An epidural catheter is also placed for more prolonged analgesia. The advantages of this technique include rapid analgesia and a low failure rate.

ANESTHESIA FOR CESAREAN DELIVERY

The anesthetic concerns related to maternal and fetal safety during a cesarean section are similar to those outlined under anesthesia for nonobstetric surgery.

Regional Anesthesia

Most cesarean sections in the United States (and increasingly around the world) are performed with spinal, epidural, or CSE anesthesia. These techniques allow the mother (and often her partner) to be alert and present for the delivery.

Regional anesthesia techniques for cesarean section are performed as described for labor analgesia. Dosing for each of the techniques must be increased to meet surgical requirements. For epidural anesthesia, approximately 20 mL of an adequate local anesthetic will provide surgical anesthesia to a T4 to T6 level. Medications commonly used include 2% lidocaine, 0.5% bupivacaine, or 3% chloroprocaine. Recently the use of 0.5% levo-bupivacaine and 0.5% to 1% ropivacaine have been described.

Lidocaine and bupivacaine are the spinal medications most commonly used for cesarean section. Administration of 60 to 80 mg of lidocaine (2% or 5%) or 10 to 15 mg of bupivacaine (0.5% to 0.75%) provides adequate anesthesia for 60 to 90 and 90 to 180 minutes, respectively. The CSE technique is used when there are concerns that the procedure might last longer than the spinal anesthetic.

The addition of a narcotic to either epidural or spinal for cesarean section improves anesthetic quality. Fentanyl (50 to 100 µg epidural, 10 to 35 µg intrathecal) or sufentanil (up to 30 µg epidural or 5 to 10 µg intrathecal) decrease maternal pain and improve satisfaction. The addition of preservative-free morphine (1 to 5 mg epidural, 100 to 300 µg intrathecal) provides postoperative analgesia for up to 24 hours.

General Anesthesia

General anesthesia for cesarean section is reserved for those instances in which there is a contraindication to regional (maternal local or systemic infection, coagulopathy, hypovolemia, or refusal), regional anesthesia is ineffective, or there is not time to administered a regional (fetal distress). Concerns related to general anesthesia for cesarean section are similar to those outlined in the section on nonobstetric surgery. Anesthesia-related maternal mortality is 17 times higher with general anesthesia than with regional anesthesia. Failed intubation is the greatest concern, occurring in as many as 1 in 250 general anesthetics. The obstetric anesthesiologist should have expertise in advanced airway skills, and backup plans should be in place in the event that the trachea cannot be successfully intubated. As with any anesthetic technique, left uterine displacement, adequate maternal hydration, and careful monitoring of maternal hemodynamics are essential.

General anesthetics may cause depression of the newborn. The degree of depression is related to the duration of intrauterine exposure. Delivery of the fetus within 5 to 10 minutes of induction decreases the incidence and severity of newborn depression.

Local Anesthesia

Though rarely used, local infiltration has been described for cesarean section.

SUMMARY

Whether caring for a pregnant patient at 18 weeks of gestation who requires an appendectomy or administering an epidural for labor analgesia, the care of the parturient is different from that of any other population. The effects of the physiologic changes of pregnancy on the response to anesthesia and concerns about fetal well-being make obstetric anesthesia a unique and interesting challenge.

SUGGESTED READINGS

Santos AC, Pederson H, Finster M. Obstetric anesthesia. In: Barash PG, Cullen BF, Stoelting RK, eds. Clinical Anesthesia. 3rd Ed. Philadelphia: Lippincott-Raven, 1997:1061-1090.

Obstetrics. In: Stoelting RK, Miller RD, eds. Basics of Anesthesia. 4th Ed. New York: Churchill Livingstone, 2000:341-363.

Chestnut DH, ed. Obstetric Anesthesia: Principles and Practice. 2nd Ed. St. Louis: Mosby, 1999.

Hughes SC, Levinson G, Rosen M, eds. Shnider and Levinson's Anesthesia for Obstetrics, 4th Ed. Philadelphia: Lippincott Williams & Wilkins, 2002.

CHAPTER 17

Pain Management

Jyotsna Nagda, MD

INTRODUCTION

Relief of pain has been a predominant concern of mankind since the beginning of recorded history and is one of the great objectives of medicine. It is the most common symptom reported to physicians, accounting for more than 80% of all patients' visits to doctors. Chronic pain affects hundreds of millions of people worldwide and alters their physical and emotional functioning, decreases their quality of life, and impairs their ability to work. As many as 80 million Americans experience chronic pain and use health services up to five times more frequently than the rest of the population. Pain accounts for approximately 25% of all sick days taken in the United States, and it is estimated that the United States spends about $90 billion annually because of chronic pain. More than 550 million workdays are lost annually secondary to chronic pain. In this age of steady cost cutting in the managed care environment, this represents an expense we can no longer afford. Yet 40% of all cancer patients, 50% of nursing home patients, 55% of postoperative patients, and 70% of patients with AIDS have unrelieved or underrelieved pain.

In October 2000 the 106th US Congress passed House Resolution 3244, which President Clinton signed into law. Title VI, Section 1603, provides for the "Decade of Pain Control and Research" to begin January 2001. Pain is now designated as a public health problem of national significance. Beginning in 2001, the Joint Commission on Accreditation of Healthcare Organizations implemented new standards to assess and treat pain. To qualify for accreditation, all facilities, including rehabilitation centers, outpatient surgical centers, hospitals and nursing homes, must identify pain in patients during initial and ongoing periodic assessments and educate patients and their families about pain management.

The word pain is originally derived from the Latin *poena*, meaning punishment. The International Association for the Study of Pain defines pain as "an unpleasant sensory and emotional experience associated with actual or potential tissue damage, or described in terms of such damage." It is both a physiologic sensation and an emotional reaction to that sensation. Viewed from an evolutionary prospective, pain is perceived as a threat or damage to one's biologic integrity and has three components: sensory discriminative, motivational affective, and cognitive evaluative.

The concepts of pain and suffering are frequently mixed and sometimes confused in spite of both being two distinct phenomena. Suffering is loosely defined as "state of severe distress associated with events that threaten the intactness of person." Pain serves a protective role by warning us of imminent or actual tissue damage. If tissue damage is unavoidable, a set of excitability changes in the peripheral and central nervous systems establish profound but reversible pain hypersensitivity in inflamed and surrounding tissue. This process avoids further damage until wound healing has occurred. In contrast, chronic pain syndromes offer no biologic advantage and cause suffering and distress.

PAIN PATHWAYS

There are two classes of afferent nerve fibers, which are responsible for communicating nociceptive information in humans. The A delta fibers are rapidly conducting myelinated fibers that conduct thermal or mechanical information at the rate of 5-30 m/sec. Pain ascribed to these fibers is characterized as sharp and pricking. C fibers are small-diameter unmyelinated fibers, which conduct impulses slowly at the rate of 0.5 to 2 m/sec and are responsible for transmission of dull pain.

At the distal end of primary afferent axons (especially A delta and C fibers) there are morphologically unique structures called nociceptors, which supply skin, subcutaneous tissue, periosteum, joints, muscles, and the viscera. They are depolarized by noxious thermal, mechanical, or chemical stimuli. Some are activated by only one type of stimulus (e.g., high-threshold mechanoreceptors) and others by more than one type (i.e., polymodal nociceptors).

Axons in A delta and C fibers carry nociceptive information to the spinal cord, or in the case of the trigeminal nerve, to the brainstem nuclei. These fibers are mainly carried through the posterior root (and in some cases by the ventral root) of the spinal cord. Nociceptive afferent fibers from skin terminate in laminae I, II, and V of the dorsal horn. Afferents from viscera, muscle, and other deep tissues end in laminae I, V, and X. Impulses are transmitted to the ascending spinal nociceptive pathways that comprise the spinothalamic, spinoreticular, spinal mesencephalic, and postsynaptic dorsal column tracts.

The spinothalamic tract crosses the midline and ascends to the opposite side of the spinal cord to project to a number of thalamic targets, which include the ventral posterolateral nucleus, posterior nuclei, the central nucleus, and the nucleus submedius. Fibers that project from the ventral posterolateral nucleus to the primary sensory cortex transmit information on the location of pain.

The spinoreticular pathway ascends on both sides of the spinal cord to the intralaminar nuclei of both right and left thalami, from which numerous projections involved in memory and emotions travel to the cingulate gyrus. Nociceptive information is processed in the cingulate cortex, periaqueductal gray matter, thalamus, lentiform nucleus, insula anterior, prefrontal cortex, inferior parietal cortex, and primary and secondary cortices.

CLASSIFICATION OF PAIN

Pain classification is based on neurophysiologic mechanism, temporal aspects, etiology, and region affected.

The neurophysiologic classification is based on the inferred mechanism of pain, which are of two types: nociceptive pain and non-nociceptive pain. The term nociceptive is applied to pain that is presumed to be maintained by continual tissue injury. Nociceptive pain results from the activation or sensitization of nociceptors in the periphery, which transduce noxious stimuli into electrochemical impulses. These impulses are then transmitted to the spinal cord and higher rostral centers within the central nervous system. Arthritic pain and acute postoperative pain are in this category. Nociceptive pain is further subdivided into somatic and visceral pain.

Non-nociceptive pain is subdivided into neuropathic and idiopathic pain. Neuropathic pain results from injury to neural structures within the peripheral or central nervous system, whereas idiopathic pain implies a wider spectrum of poorly understood pain states.

The temporal classification of pain is based on the duration of symptoms and is usually divided into acute and chronic. The etiologic classification is based on the primary process (e.g., cancer pain, arthritis pain).

Acute Pain

Acute pain signifies the presence of a noxious stimulus that produces actual tissue damage or possesses the potential to do so. The sensation of acute pain implies the presence of an intact nervous system and is usually associated with autonomic hyperactivity (e.g., hypertension, tachycardia, sweating, vasoconstriction). A common definition of acute pain is "the normal, predicted physiological response to an adverse chemical, thermal or mechanical stimulus, associated with surgery, trauma and acute illness." Acute pain is usually short lived.

Inadequate pain relief in the acute postoperative period leads to numerous adverse effects including activation of the neuroendocrine response, stressful changes in the cardiovascular system and coagulation, impairment of pulmonary and gastrointestinal functions, sleep disturbance, impaired ambulation, and the risk of immobility. It also delays recovery and discharge from the hospital, leading to a greater and more expensive use of health-care resources.

Pharmacologic management of acute pain usually includes nonopioid analgesics (e.g., acetaminophen and nonsteroidal anti-inflammatory agents) and systemically or neuroaxially administered opioid analgesics. Systemic opioids may be given orally, intramuscularly, intravenously, transdermally, rectally, or via the subcutaneous route. Intravenous opioids may be given as intermittent bolus doses, as a continuous infusion, or through a patient-controlled analgesia (PCA) pump. PCA allows the patient to self-administer opioids intravenously at a prescribed interval. The PCA pump is a microprocessor-controlled device, which allows the clinician to choose an incremental dose, lock-out interval, maximum dose per hour, and optional basal rate. Neuroaxial opioids may be given epidurally or intrathecally.

REGIONAL AND LOCAL ANALGESIA OR ANESTHESIA FOR ACUTE PAIN

Direct injection of local anesthetic drugs close to a peripheral nerve, major nerve trunks, nerve root, or intra-articular space may produce analgesia by blocking afferent impulses. Neural blockade with local anesthetics and opioids is a very safe and effective method for managing postoperative pain. An epidural catheter can be placed close to the dermatomes approximating the site of surgical injury, and an infusion of a combination of a local anesthetic and an opioid can provide segmental analgesia in the perioperative period. Intrathecal opioids may also be used.

Benefits of epidural analgesia include decreased pain during mobilization, earlier return of bowel function after abdominal surgery, decreased pulmonary complications, shorter time in the intensive care unit, and reduced length of hospital stay.

Nonpharmacologic interventions for the treatment of acute pain include cryotherapy or heat, which may reduce pain when applied to the operative and perioperative site. In addition, physical and occupational therapies may help decrease pain, as well as speed recovery and increase the patient's function.

Chronic Pain

Nearly one third of the people in the United States suffer from chronic pain at some point in their lives. Recent scientific evidence points toward chronic pain being a destructive disease process that creates pathologic changes in the central and peripheral nervous systems. Pain that extends beyond the usual period of healing in the absence of ongoing pathology is considered to be chronic pain. Traditionally, chronic pain is subdivided into malignant pain (i.e., pain associated with cancer) and nonmalignant pain (as from other syndromes unrelated to cancer).

ASSESSMENT OF CHRONIC PAIN

The assessment of chronic pain requires a complete history and comprehensive physical examination. A complete and detailed history of the pain should include a description of location, intensity, character, exacerbating and relieving factors, and its possible mechanisms. Several self-reporting scales (e.g., the Verbal Descriptor Scale, Numerical Rating Scale, Visual Analog Scale, Faces Pain Rating Scale) have been used to assess pain. There are several multidimensional instruments, which are used to assess complex pain, including the McGill Pain Questionnaire, the Brief Pain Inventory, and the Dartmouth Pain Questionnaire.

A complete physical examination should include a general physical examination followed by neurologic, musculoskeletal, and mental status assessments. Complete assessment of pain includes the analysis of the psychological aspects of pain and the effects of pain on the patient's behavior and emotional stability.

Diagnostic neural blockade with local anesthetics (including somatic and autonomic blockade) may be useful in determining the site and etiology of chronic pain.

MANAGEMENT OF CHRONIC PAIN

Practical goals of chronic pain management include maximal reduction in pain, helping the patient to cope with any residual pain, and increasing the patient's functional capacity. It is important to realize that just taking the pain away does not instantly eliminate the environmental, cognitive, behavioral, emotional, biochemical, neurophysiologic, and social consequences that the patient's pain has produced. Multiple modalities, such as the combined use of neural blockade, medications, or rehabilitative therapies should be considered when analgesia is no longer attained with a single technique. A comprehensive multidisciplinary approach may reduce the potential for adverse effects arising from either escalating frequency or dosage levels of a single modality.

PHARMACOLOGIC MANAGEMENT

For most chronic pain of nonmalignant origin, nonsteroidal anti-inflammatory drugs (NSAIDs) and acetaminophen are useful analgesics. NSAIDs are potent inhibitors of cyclooxygenase enzymes, which convert arachidonic acid to prostaglandins. Two types of cyclooxygenase enzymes have been identified, COX-1 and COX-2. Drugs that selectively inhibit COX-2 (e.g., rofecoxib and celecoxib) provide analgesia and inflammatory activity with less organ toxicity than COX-1 inhibitors. Acetaminophen has minimal anti-inflammatory action at its analgesic potency. It has an excellent safety profile with respect to gastroduodenal mucosa and platelet function but may cause hepatotoxicity at chronic doses higher than 6 g/day. Acetaminophen and NSAIDs share a ceiling dose effect for analgesia.

Neuropathic pain is best treated with antidepressants and antiepileptics. Antidepressants work by inhibiting the reuptake of serotonin and norepinephrine in the descending inhibitory tracts of the spinal cord. These drugs include tricyclic antidepressants and selective serotonin reuptake inhibitors. Antiepileptics suppress spontaneous neuronal firing through membrane-stabilizing effects and seem to be most effective in managing pain states that have a prominent lancinating component. Carbamazepine has a well-established efficacy in the management of trigeminal neuralgia. Gabapentin has demonstrated efficacy in reducing pain in diabetic neuropathy and in postherpetic neuralgia. Lamotrigine, topiramate, and various other anticonvulsants have also been used for chronic neuropathic pain.

Baclofen, an analog of the inhibitory neurotransmitter γ-aminobutyric acid has been used both orally and intrathecally in the management of chronic pain. It is also used intrathecally in the management of severe spasticity of spinal cord origin.

α_2-Adrenergic agonists such as clonidine and tizanidine are also used in the management of chronic pain.

Tramadol is a unique drug used for analgesic purposes in several chronic pain states. Its mechanism of action is mediated by both μ opiate receptor stimulation and inhibition of reuptake of norepinephrine and serotonin.

Opioids are a necessary and effective component of management of chronic nonmalignant pain in some patients. Individual opioids vary in their potency and degree of adverse effects. Morphine sulphate is the prototypical opioid drug. The molecular mechanism causing analgesia remains the same for all opiates: they bind to G protein-coupled peripheral and central opioid receptors with subsequent inhibition of adenylate cyclase, activation of potassium channels, and inhibition of voltage-gated calcium channels, all of which decrease neuronal excitability. The five subtypes of opioid receptors include μ, κ, δ, σ, and ϵ. The relatively pure opioid agonists include morphine, codeine, oxycodone, levorphanol, meperidine, fentanyl, and methadone. The mixed agonist–antagonist drugs include pentazocine, butorphanol, and buprenorphine. Analgesic therapy with long-acting opioids offers convenient dosage intervals that reach safe, effective steady-state levels. Adverse effects of opioids include constipation, nausea, vomiting, sedation, confusion, respiratory depression, and development of tolerance. Table 17-1 describes pharmacokinetic data for some commonly used opioids (see Chapter 4).

Table 17.1   Pharmacokinetics of Opioids

Opioids	Route	Equianalgesic Dose (mg)	Peak (hr)	Duration (hr)	Half-life (hr)
Morphine	IM	10–15	0.5–1.0	3–5	2.0–3.5
	PO	30–60	1.0–1.5	3–4	
	SC	30–60	2	8–12	
Codeine	IM	120	0.5–1.0	4–6	3
PO	30–200			3–4	
Hydro-codone	PO	10	1	4–6	3.8–4.5
Hydro-morphone	IM	1–2	0.5–1.0	3–4	2–3
	PO	2–4	1.5–2.0	4–6	
Oxycodone	PO	30	1	4–6	2–3
Levorphanol	IM	2	0.5–1.0	5–8	12–16
	PO	4	1.5–2.0		
Methadone	IM	8–10	0.5–1.0	4–8	15–30
	PO	20	1.5–2.0	4–12	
Propoxy-phene	PO	32–65	2–2.5	4–6	3.5
Meperidine	IM	75–100	0.5–1.0	2–3	2.5
	PO	200–300	1–2	2–3	

IM, intramuscular; PO, per os (orally); SC, subcutaneous route.

CANCER PAIN

Thirty percent to 50% of cancer patients in active treatment and 60% to 90% of patients with advanced malignancy report significant pain. Multiple causes and sites are common, with up to 81% of patients reporting two or more types of pain and 34% reporting three. Bone pain is the most common, followed by pain from tumor infiltration of nerve and hollow viscera. In addition, pain associated with cancer therapy occurs in 15% to 25% of patients undergoing surgery, radiation therapy, or chemotherapy. In children that figure is much higher, with up to 60% of patients reporting procedure-associated pain.

Palliative Care

The World Health Organization defines palliative care as the active, total care of patients whose disease is not responsive to the curative treatment. The goal of such care is achievement of the best quality of life for the patients and their families. Hospice refers to a program of care for terminally ill patients. Most hospice programs are home-care based, whereas palliative care units are within or affiliated with hospitals or other inpatient facilities.

Pharmacologic Management

As elucidated in the World Health Organization guidelines, pain medications are to be administered in a three-step ladder approach according to the intensity and pathophysiology of symptoms and individual requirements (Fig. 17-1). For patients with mild pain, the recommended baseline drugs are NSAIDs. Patients with moderate to severe pain usually require an opioid agent.

There is also a rapidly growing category of adjuvant analgesic drugs that were not specifically developed for pain control but that have analgesic properties and can be used in conjunction with NSAIDs or opioids. These include antidepressants (both tricyclic antidepressants and serotonin reuptake inhibitors), neuroleptics, corticosteroids, anticonvulsants, and psychostimulants.

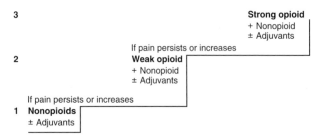

FIGURE 17-1. The World Health Organization analgesic ladder.

OTHER PAIN MANAGEMENT MODALITIES

Interventional pain management includes peripheral and central neural blocking techniques, sympathetic nervous system blocking techniques, continuous epidural or plexus anesthesia, and chemical, surgical, and thermal neurolysis. More-invasive interventions include neuromodulatory techniques such as spinal cord stimulation, peripheral nerve stimulation, deep brain stimulation, and the implantation of pumps (for continuous intrathecal infusion of opioids alone or in combinations with local anesthetics, or α_2-adrenergic agents like clonidine or centrally acting medications like baclofen). Intrathecal infusion is also used to treat various conditions with spasticity including multiple sclerosis, spinal cord trauma, poststroke rigidity, and cerebral palsy.

Physical Therapy

Physical modalities used to treat pain directly and indirectly include cold application, radiant heat, ultrasound, diathermy, microwave, and laser.

Exercise has long been a fundamental tool in the treatment of musculoskeletal pain and is one of the commonly prescribed remedies for patients with back pain. The objectives are decreasing pain, strengthening weak muscles, decreasing mechanical stress on spinal structures, improving fitness level to prevent injury, stabilizing hypermobile spinal segments, improving posture, and improving mobility.

Occupational therapy focuses on body mechanics, and helps patients to return to more normal levels of activity in household chores, work, and leisure.

Emotional and Behavioral Management of Pain

Techniques for emotional and behavioral management of pain are oriented toward reducing pain and pain-related disability, treating comorbid psychiatric illness, increasing perception of control and self-efficacy, decreasing maladaptive behavior, and developing specific coping skills. These techniques include relaxation techniques, hypnotic techniques, biofeedback, and cognitive-behavioral therapies.

Acupuncture has been used as a treatment of pain for thousands of years. Although scientific data have not been able to support many of its diverse claims, there is evidence that acupuncture may be effective in relieving certain types of pain.

SUMMARY

Pain management is a complex problem that provides the clinician with a difficult challenge in medicine's present state of flux. Effective application of the available knowledge and therapies can reduce prolonged suffering and disability and thus improve the quality of life for millions of patients with pain. A comprehensive pain management program that provides a coordinated, goal-oriented, interdisciplinary approach can improve the functional status of patients with pain and decrease their dependence on the health-care system.

SUGGESTED READINGS

Benzon H, Raja S, Borsook D, Molloy RE, Strichartz G. Essentials of Pain Medicine and Regional Anesthesia. New York: Churchill Livingstone, 1999.

Ballantyne JC, Fishman S, Abdi S. The Massachusetts General Hospital Handbook of Pain Management. Philadelphia: Lippincott Williams & Wilkins, 2001.

Loeser JD, Butler SH, Chapman CR, Turk DC. Bonica's Management of Pain. 3rd Ed. Philadelphia: Lippincott Williams & Wilkins, 2001.

Cousins MJ, Bridenbaugh PO. Neural Blockade in Anesthesia and Pain Management. Philadelphia: Lippincott Williams & Wilkins, 1998.

Index

Page numbers in *italics* denote figures; those followed by a t denote tables.